Going to the Dogs

ALSO BY M. LOUISE HEYDT

Divine Rainbow, Nature as Spiritual Teacher
 (First Place—New Mexico Book Awards 2007)

Going to the Dogs

An Incredible True Story

M. Louise Heydt

SUNSTONE
PRESS

SANTA FE

Sunstone books may be purchased for educational, business, or sales promotional use.
For information please write: Special Markets Department, Sunstone Press,
P.O. Box 2321, Santa Fe, New Mexico 87504-2321.

Book and Cover design › Vicki Ahl
Body typeface › Contantia
Printed on acid-free paper

Library of Congress Cataloging-in-Publication Data

Heydt, M. Louise, 1942-
 Going to the dogs : an incredible true story / by M. Louise Heydt.
    pages cm
  ISBN 978-0-86534-952-0 (softcover : alkaline paper)
  1. Dogs--Behavior. 2. Dogs--Psychology. 3. Human-animal relationships. 4.
Human-animal communication. 5. Families--United States. 6. Spirituality--Unit-
ed States. 7. Heydt, M. Louise, 1942- 8. Dog owners--United States--Biography. I.
Title.
  SF433.H48 2013
  636.7'089689142--dc23

                        2013010591

WWW.SUNSTONEPRESS.COM
SUNSTONE PRESS / POST OFFICE BOX 2321 / SANTA FE, NM 87504-2321 /USA
(505) 988-4418 / ORDERS ONLY (800) 243-5644 / FAX (505) 988-1025

For

Alan
and
Zuma

"Every animal and human are put together for a reason."

—Laura's cat, Joey

FOREWORD

In this book, Louise takes us on a spiritual journey of discovering the inner depths of our relationships with animals. We follow her and her animals through illness, death, dying, surviving chaos, and the magical joy of experiencing living with our compassionate animals. Many of us have regrets for the way we dealt with certain situations involving animals in our past. Louise is brutally honest with her readers about her shortcomings. Through this extraordinary account, we learn that we can make amends with our animals. This is not only healing for our pets but also for us.

Following this family, we learn to grow, flourish, trust, and be strong while making decisions that anyone would dread. We witness that our animals not only are understanding of our difficult decisions, but also are often an integral part of making these decisions. Our animals are communicating with us all the time. Sometimes we consciously know what they are saying and other times it is unconscious yet still happening.

I am a professional animal communicator / pet psychic. This means I can telepathically talk to animals. I can ask or tell them anything. There is no limit to the consciousness of animals. We see through my communications with Louise's pets that animals can take on many voices. One moment they can sound innocent like a child and then later offer advice like a wise sage. We see them scared of illness and death but once they understand the process they open their hearts and trust. They ground us in the present by asking for certain foods, to be read to and for walks in nature. They tell Louise to stretch and drink tea in order to be more centered and calm. They open our eyes to different realms by talking about visits from spiritual beings, deceased loved ones on the other side, and by telling us what happens to them after death. We learn that a golden thread always connects us and even death does not break the extraordinary bond we have with our animals.

This is a powerful story of elevating consciousness. While reading this wonderful book you will cry, laugh, be in wonder, forgive yourself and grow with Louise and her animal family. Once finished your heart will be open. Undoubtedly your life and relationships with all animals will change in remarkable ways.

—Laura Stinchfield

PREFACE

The words that Genji, Rasa, Tara, and Kundun speak are unaltered. These are their direct quotes as translated by Laura Stinchfield from the visual images she received from them into the verbal language we understand as humans. I, of course, have added punctuation and woven their image-words into the story as I know it from our lives together.

Sometimes they randomly string completely different and unrelated subjects and/or ideas together in the same thought-expression. I have left these untouched except for adding punctuation for clarity. The reader may be surprised by how their individual personalities immediately come forward based in each one's "voice" and perspective.

It is my hope as the author that the reader will realize by the end of the book that our companion animals have thoughts and feelings, as indeed so do wild animals, and that this will completely change the point of view that animals are inferior to humans. I wonder if we aren't inferior for not being able to understand them. Our animal companions rely on their human caretakers for everything—food, water, shelter, love, understanding, and being kept safe. They also do not miss a thing—intentions, actions emotions or even thoughts.

It is also my hope that the reader will grasp the lifelong effects that abuse has on animals. Tara's abuse was the most insidious kind perpetrated by employees at her own home when I was out of town, or even just gone to do errands—her home where she should have been safe. The gradual revelation of this violence and betrayal had its effect on me as much as Tara. It created a deep wound that we share.

Our story spans thirteen years, however the conversations take place over a period of four years. In that time Laura, Genji, Rasa, Tara, Kundun, and I had over sixty conversations. Sinister, dark situations were revealed. We shared humorous, laughable moments. I discovered that Tara is a poet. I had to acknowledge my own character flaws and work on myself to overcome them. My relationship with all of them deepened as I gained more insight into their heart-minds, what in Chinese is called *shin,* and is not considered two separate aspects as it is in western thought.

And yes, animals go to Heaven when they die. The reader will have a glimpse of what Heaven is like, and will probably be very surprised. As a result of my mystical experiences in nature prior to this, I had begun to believe that Heaven, or the Other Side, or whatever name you give it—is an alternate reality that exists simultaneously. After these conversations, I am convinced it is.

Finally, this is at its heart, a compelling story of a family being confronted with aging, illness, death and dying, as well as courage and hopefulness in the face of cruel abuse, and compassionate loving kindness in the practice of life.

ACKNOWLEDGEMENTS

The man in the blue truck from Lower Colonias who abandoned his puppy on the side of the road—thank you—one of the best dogs I've ever had.

Breeder Tom Turner from Georgia, whose matchmaking between Sweet-Tea and T-Bo created my Catahoula girls. Thank you for convincing me to take the last magical dog left in the litter as well as the one I chose from a photo.

Veterinarians Dr. Nicci Quinn, Dr. Janis Shinkawa, Dr. Jill Muraoka Lim, Dr. Katherine Byrne, and all of the excellent staff at Buena Animal Hospital in Ventura for expert diagnosis, compassion and care.

Oncology veterinarian, Dr. Alice Villalobos, and her excellent staff for the miracle of cancer cure and giving grateful animal owners more time with their beloved pets.

Acupuncture veterinarians Dr. Karen Martin and Dr. Liz Fernandez for keeping my dogs walking when it didn't seem possible.

Horse veterinarian, Dr. Ellice Rubin, for chiropractic treatments, diagnostic explanations and good preventative advice.

Catherine Gould-Stern PhD, Steve Matzkin DC, Sherry D. Gaber DC.

Dr. Kathleen Ayl, pet loss recovery specialist.

Suzanne, Sandra, Chef Max, and the exceptional staff at Suzanne's Restaurant in Ojai where I eat lunch regularly, am allowed to customize everything on the menu, and have a captive audience with the saga of my animals. This is my extended family and support group.

Laura Stinchfield without whose skills and wisdom there would be no story to tell. Thank you from all of us with all of our hearts. We love you.

Kaethe, Marilyn, Cassidy and RuthAnne for listening, loving and believing.

1

Snowflakes drift through the landscape like giant butterflies, a kaleidoscope of white, earth and sky inseparable. It is night and the only light is the reflection off the snow that completely surrounds us. I am walking between my two sisters taller than both of them. Our feet crunch on the ground. It is the only sound. My sister on my left begins to rotate her shoulders and shrink toward the ground. Suddenly she is Wuli, furry black Chow prancing happily through the snow, tail wagging. In her mouth is the bright green, fuzzy sheep doll that belongs to Tara. In an instant Wuli becomes Rasa who shreds Tara's dolly. I wake, sit up and reach out to touch Rasa and Tara who sleep on my bed —my special girls, crazy Catahoula Leopard Hounds, now nine years old.

I replay the dream over and over in my mind. Wuli, what are you trying to tell me? Is something going to happen to Tara because it's her doll and it's demolished? Or is something going to happen to Rasa because she destroyed it? At the time I have no idea how prophetic the dream will be, or what a journey my dogs, my horse and I will end up pursuing. What I do know is that ever since my precious black Chow died in my arms in a tipi at Moon Dragon Ranch ten years ago, she has revealed in dreams future events concerning my four-legged friends.

In July I take Rasa and Tara with me to visit my sister who lives in Napa. They love her ranch. Catahoulas are hunting fools. They love to chase, they love to bark. The Louisiana Catahoula is named for both its place of origin and the unique leopard spotted pattern on some. This pattern is associated with the merle gene, which also causes blue and green color eyes. They can have each eye be a different color, which is called split-eyes. Both Rasa and Tara sport the leopard pattern. Rasa has blue eyes and Tara has what the breeders call yellow eyes—a dark amber color reminiscent of a wolf. The breed is a mix of red wolves, and fighting dogs brought to America by Hernando DeSoto which included mastiffs and greyhounds. After DeSoto's defeat the dogs were abandoned, roamed freely and bred with each other as well as with red wolves.

Native Americans called them "wolf dogs" and used them for hunting. The French brought the "Bas Rouge" breed and bred them to the "wolf dogs." They are internationally famous as wild pig hunters. They are fearless, intelligent, and tough. They are protective, territorial, and independent thinkers. They need a job and a lot of exercise.

At my sister's property in Wild Horse Valley there are horses, trucks, carts, coyotes, wild pigs, and all kinds of fabulous things to bark at and chase up and down the fence surrounding a yard behind the house. Best of all there is a lawn, which I don't have. They roll and roll for the sheer pleasure of it, run, and bark like the exuberant dogs they are having the perfect holiday. My other sister arrives to visit as well, bringing my niece and three great nephews. One day while I'm there I notice a round swollen looking lump on Rasa's thigh. My sister's yard is full of bees, so I dismiss it as a bee sting. After returning home, I think that the lump has disappeared. Because Catahoulas are black, blue and spotted it is difficult to see things on their bodies. At the end of July the light in the kitchen touches her hair just right, and she is lying at just the right angle. "Oh my God, there is that round lump on her thigh!" It is obviously not a bee sting.

I immediately call Buena Animal Hospital in Ventura where I have been taking the dogs since I moved to California less than a year ago. There is a team of three outstanding women vets, two from University of California Davis, and one from Colorado State University in Fort Collins—both excellent veterinarian schools. There is also a friendly, compassionate group of young staff members who never seem to wear out. We arrive for Rasa's appointment the next day. After aspirating the lump, Dr. Nicci sits down next to me in the waiting room. She is young, has dark hair, an athletic body, and loves her work, which she performs with much compassion and skill.

"It is a mast cell skin cancer tumor. We need to operate tomorrow morning."

She hands me some information to read, the estimate for the cost of the surgery to sign, and sends us home. My heart slips down to my toes.

2

I had moved from my two hundred acre ranch in Pecos, New Mexico to two acres in Oak View, California. I traded in my little log house and most of my belongings in storage for a Mediterranean style house in a California live oak grove fifteen minutes from the ocean. Rasa, Tara, Kundun, and Pecos made the move in a filled up Toyota SUV. Pecos, mortified yellow tabby with greenish eyes and freckles on his pink nose, traveled in a fairly roomy canvas small dog crate. Although I had food, dishes, water, little aluminum trays for disposable litter boxes, and litter, he never ate, drank, pooped, or peed for two and one-half days of travel. This probably qualified as one of the worst experiences in his life. He was seventeen years old when we left New Mexico. I had contemplated having him euthanized and leaving him behind in my pet cemetery at the ranch, but I didn't have the heart to make that decision. I had adopted him at the age of three months old from the shelter in Santa Fe, and for better or for worse he was coming with us. I am weary of having a cat. I hate the litter box, the stench of it, and burning incense every morning. Years before Pecos had fallen off the ladder to the loft and ruptured the disc in his back just in front of his tail. His hindquarters sank lower and lower as he aged until he walked on his hind legs to his elbows. He wobbled and sometimes fell over.

Pecos was a hunter. When he was young he would hunt mice outdoors all night. In the morning the mice would be neatly lined up on the doormat with all of the heads facing the door and the tails going the opposite direction. Being a very neat person, I was impressed with this display of extreme organization. He would drag rabbits as large as himself onto the deck. When he stopped hunting the house became overrun with mice and rats. I was killing them every night in glue traps, and baited mouse traps. They chewed into the corn-based litter bags and dog food bags. I began to store everything in hard plastic screw-top containers. Then they neurotically chewed on the plastic lids. They were in the ceiling and in the fireplace rock work. They scrambled through the cupboard filled with pots, pans, and small appliances, as well as the gas stove top. They were so brazen they scampered across the rooms right in front of the dogs. The Pecos wood rats are the largest rats of all. They are handsome with big ears that are round, a white chest and tawny fur. I set a rat trap on the front porch to try to catch the rat that was chewing a hole into the overhang and running through the ceiling in my bedroom. After I was in bed and asleep, there was a loud thwak!, and much to my horror thumping, clacking and banging as well. I got up and turned on the porch light. At least four feet from where I placed the trap was a rat as big as the trap, on its back in the trap, caught by the neck. He had managed to move himself in the trap that far before he died.

I began to appreciate how Pecos had kept the house rodent-free, and I became annoyed with him for getting old and so non-functional. How could he just sleep on the sofa all night and let these rats and mice take over? I'd never had a cat live so long, and I'd never relied on a cat so much to hunt. Of course I hated for him to kill birds, but he did quit hunting them eventually.

So, Pecos made it to California. He has a nice laundry room where he spends the night. He has a little snuggly day-glo green, round bed in the kitchen, and he likes to lie in a chair outside in the courtyard on warm days. He becomes thinner and thinner. It is hard to find him food he likes to eat. He trashes the laundry room every night. Before I can make tea or feed the dogs, I have to clean up his mess. He falls over in the cat box, because he can't stand on three legs to use one leg to cover up his poop. Litter and poop stick to his fur which is messy, and which I have to clean off, and it annoys me early in the morning. He can't help it, but I can't deal with it. I don't seem to possess unconditional love, and I am bothered by this.

3

When Rasa comes home from her surgery she is confined to the kitchen with a plastic cone-shaped collar around her neck. This is to keep her from licking or biting her incision site. It was an aggressive tumor, and a cancerous tumor has to have a three centimeter margin around it removed. Therefore she has a six inch incision on her right thigh with a lot of underlying tissue now gone. Being confined to the kitchen, Rasa wants to let me know how unhappy she is. So, she pees and poops in multiple places—on bare satillo tiles, on area rugs. I move out the rugs and place potty pads everywhere at night before I go to bed. To her credit, she self-trains to use the potty pads at the age of ten years old.

In the morning I am confronted with the kitchen mess and let Rasa outside. Kundun sleeps in an all-weather synthetic rattan crate, which he is now attempting to chew his way out of. If I leave him out of his crate at night he pees on the rock fireplace. He rushes outside with Rasa. Then I open the laundry room door and I'm confronted with Pecos' mess—the stench, litter everywhere. He opens drawers to let me know he is unhappy. He climbs in the bottom one to hide. Tara very wisely stays upstairs in bed until the coast is clear then comes downstairs to go outside after the kitchen and laundry room are clean. I do all of this before my first cup of tea and I am not happy.

After one week I realize I can't cope. I find Cindy and Cat Vacations in Ventura and check Pecos in for a month.

Rasa has a funny way of maneuvering around with her collar. She has a swagger to her walk, and this makes the collar-cone move from side to side, which crashes into whatever is near her. She barrels through any obstacle clearing a path in front of her. This apparition scares Tara, and I am continuously standing by Rasa to push the sides in toward her head so she can get through doors without taking the door with her. Before two weeks have gone by and the date for Rasa to get her stitches removed approaches, Rasa and Kundun decide to have an adventure, jump off a six foot high wall into a courtyard between the dog yard and the driveway. The gate is accidently left open, which I'm certain they notice, and off they run to explore the front yard area and the oak covered hillside beyond. They immediately find a rabbit to chase into the bushes before I realize what is happening. My fear ever since moving is that they will run into the street, chase cars and get hit, because they know nothing about the reality of a real street with fast moving vehicles. I call them and they come running back, however when I see Rasa I realize that her incision has opened, is oozing and on closer inspection smells really terrible.

A trip to see Dr. Nicci reveals that the cancer is activated. Rasa has a second surgery the following morning and this time most of her thigh muscle is removed to get the three centimeter margin. I feel desperate. My nerves are tangled. Sleep consists of lying awake in bed all night. My beloved dog might not survive this nightmare. I am reacting by being upset at everything. My world is collapsing around me.

I call Laura Stinchfield, the local animal communicator, who has a column called "The Pet Psychic" in the Ojai Valley Newspaper which I enjoy reading. We make an appointment for her to come to my home and talk to my dogs. My intention is to let Rasa know why she has had two major surgeries, and is confined to the kitchen all night every night for weeks and weeks after sleeping on my bed for seven years.

Laura arrives and we all gather in the kitchen. Laura has clear blue eyes that reflect her joy of being in the presence of animals. Her long light brown hair is pulled back from her face giving her a youthful look. She wears no make-up which she doesn't need. Her inner beauty radiates outward including all in its enthusiasm. There are Rasa, Tara, her full sister and fellow wild hound, and Kundun, the big-hearted, tail wagging, brindle pit bull mix I rescued as a puppy. Rasa and Tara are ten years old after celebrating their birthday in August, and Kundun is almost nine years old. Laura engages Rasa first. She gets eye contact up close then talks to her without sound. Her mouth is moving subtly, but the communication is with images. What fascinates me is how Rasa moves right up next to her with full eye contact to engage in a conversation. I think I know my dogs fairly well, but this opens up a dimension I am completely missing.

"Tara gave me cancer!" Rasa exclaims.

"Tara is a very spiritual dog. See how her eyes bulge?"

"She is named after the Tibetan Buddhist deity, Tara," I comment.

When Laura says this, Kundun asks, "Do my eyes bulge?"

They all want to know, "Why can't Mom communicate with us like Laura?"

"Communicate with music," Rasa suggests to me.

Tara now wants to go outside so I open the door. She lays on the bed right outside the kitchen door which is glass, so we can see her. Suddenly Laura turns toward her, then opens the door and goes outside where she squats down next to Tara in her bed. They seem to have a lengthy conversation.

"The man with the boots kicked me in the head. Everything looks like a cracked mirror. It's hard for me to trust anyone."

I nearly weep. Suddenly I understand what had happened while I was traveling in Burma in 2004, four years earlier in November. This explained the scar next to Tara's eye. It explained the blood all over her bed in her crate which had been turned over to hide it, which I didn't see until I washed dog bedding. My caretaker, Jake, had reached into her crate to grab her by the collar to force her out, and she had bitten him—this much he had told me. But by now I knew that Jake lied and told half-truths. Now I understood why Tara had been completely terrified of Jake.

While I was traveling in Burma, Tara sent me a stream of vivid images of her being hit in the head. They came day and night. It was so unbearable that I closed my mind to her for the remainder of my journey. I had no idea what she was trying to tell me. Unfortunately I did not understand animal communication at the time. What a different message than what she had sent me when I was in Burma the first time four years earlier in 2000. She stuck her nose in my ear and kissed me. It was so real I woke up and felt my ear expecting it to be wet.

The day I returned home from my trip to Burma I noticed that I was out of cat food. I thought that I would take Rasa and Tara for a ride in the car to the grocery store twenty miles away. It was late afternoon and cold. I walked out the door with both dogs on leashes. Before I could close the door they started fighting. Their blue leashes became tangled. I dropped one leash, and unfortunately it was Tara's. She ran from the porch up the valley into the forest, the leash dragging behind her. I immediately put Rasa in the house, and went to the Pecos Village general store five miles from home to buy the cat food. When I returned I gathered up a flashlight, water, and dressed for hours of searching at night for a dog whose leash was probably caught somewhere in the steep, rugged, forested canyon where we lived. The chances of finding her before a mountain lion, pack of coyotes or a bobcat were slim.

As I left the house Tara came trotting up—no leash. I saw that her old leather collar had torn where the ring held the leash. The ring and the leash hooked to it were gone. The next day I told Jake about these strange images and this event. That is when he told me that he had reached into her crate to get her out and she bit him. Then he took her on a walk and she wouldn't go back into the house. She was out in the cold weather too scared to go into the house. He fed her on the porch. Finally he thought of opening the gate into the yard and she went in on her own after three days and nights. I didn't like his story. He had a history of lying to me. You don't force an animal to do something, especially Tara. I had explained endlessly that the crate was her safe place. Well, not now. I took the collars off the dogs so they couldn't be grabbed. I was furious.

Lanky and tall, Jake had friendly eyes that were a hazel color. He was puppy-like in his enthusiasm to work. He never thought it was cold because his family came from North Dakota. So, he worked outdoors all year in all weather. He was a hard worker and he loved my land. He and Karen were very religious and went to church all day every Sunday. They had no concept of water conservation or recycling. Jake moved too quickly and jerkily around the horses which scared them. I think he learned a lot from me, but unfortunately not to stop lying.

"I was a snake. I lied all the time to my parents."

He lied to me about my animals in his care that had no voice—until now.

Laura and I sit in our chairs looking at each other silently for a few moments.

"Obviously you can't have one conversation, can you?" I conclude. "I'll call you."

4

My neighbor recommends an oncology veterinarian in Los Angeles who she had taken her white German Shepard, Sundance, to when he got a tumor on his foot, "His tumor never came back."

I have never heard of an oncology vet. I call to make an appointment with Dr. Alice Villalobos, and am happy to find out that on Wednesdays she is in Woodland Hills, which is much closer to Ventura than Hermosa Beach.

In early October Rasa and I drive south on the 101 to Woodland Hills. Dr. Villalobos' office there is an emergency veterinarians' clinic that is unused during weekdays. We sit in the waiting room. Other dogs and owners are waiting, checking out, or on their way in to see Dr. Alice. It is much like a people doctor's waiting room. An extremely concerned gay couple has their golden lab that they are constantly touching and fussing over. A woman in tears has a cat in a crate. I am attempting to keep Rasa next to me and away from other dogs. She is an alpha female, other dog aggressive, and territorial. I am trying to keep anything from happening, because she doesn't growl—she just lunges with her mouth open. If she arrives to an empty room, then it is her room and needs to be kept clear of intruders. If she arrives to a full room, then it needs to be cleared out so it becomes her room. This creates problems everywhere we go.

Rasa is weighed and we are ushered into a small treatment room. Dr. Alice enters the room with a swirl of her white coat. She has sparkly, engaging dark eyes, dark hair, looks slender and fit, and seems excited to see a Catahoula.

"Treating a Catahoula is like treating a truck!" she announces.

"They are tough dogs, but extremely sensitive," I add.

"This is going to be her regimen. She will have chemotherapy every week for ten weeks. She will take supplements to boost her immune system and get anti-oxidants. There is something for vomiting, and something for diarrhea if she reacts to the chemo. She needs to take pepsid every day, and she will take prednisone. She has a sister? Feed her all of the supplements as well."

Rasa is ushered out for her first weekly chemo-treatment. Dr. Alice hands me a folder filled with information about mast cell skin cancer, all of the supplements, and about her. I am given a calendar with which day she takes what, and handed a gigantic invoice. I look around the waiting room at dogs in various states of health, and at their people looking hopeful. I put Rasa in the car, return to pay the bill, and pick up the large bag of drugs and supplements. On the drive home I begin to realize just what is ahead of us on the path to recovery. That night I pray to be able to enjoy and love Rasa one more year.

At first I am so confused with her chart that I have to fill in the days of the weeks and draw lines with color marker pens to try to keep it straight. She takes an oral chemo capsule called leukeran every other day. You are supposed to use rubber gloves to handle it, but I soon give up and simply wash my hands afterwards. She takes prednisone with it every other day. She takes over the counter pepsid every day. I learn quickly to start using the generic which costs less. Those all stay on the kitchen counter. In the laundry room where I feed the dogs are the supplements, except for the one that has to be refrigerated.

Wednesdays are my regular days to go to the stable and ride Genji. For ten weeks Wednesdays are spent driving the 101 to Woodland Hills. On the return trips I begin to take random exits to try to find a place to have lunch. In this way I learn about the area, and in the process find a wonderful organic restaurant in Westlake Village. One criterion for somewhere to eat is a place to park in the shade for Rasa. This has beautiful huge sycamore trees in the parking lot.

"Don't let Rasa get hot. Mast cells love heat," Dr. Alice warns me.

Meanwhile, Genji is not seeing me on Wednesdays. Rasa's situation is taking a lot of my time and energy, and becomes emotionally draining. Sometimes on weekends I can't find the energy to get to the stable, so I see Genji less and less.

In mid-October I go to Los Angeles to visit my daughter for the weekend. I board Kundun and Tara at a kennel in Santa Paula, where they had stayed previously. Rasa comes with me so that I can take care of her with her complicated regimen. She has a wonderful outing in the Hollywood Hills. She takes over my daughter's English Mastiff, Crush's, cushy bed that he never uses, and as we find out later, she barked out on the deck the entire time we were at dinner and a movie. This is now her territory.

I pick up Kundun and Tara and take all three to have baths at Grooming by Amanda in Oak View. I don't notice anything wrong with Tara, but that night when she gets up to turn around and lie back down, she keeps lying closer and closer to Rasa who sleeps on the foot of the bed. I don't realize what is happening until at dawn she flops on top of Rasa. Rasa growls and starts to attack her. Awake now I sit up and bark, "What is going on here?"

I get up, take Rasa downstairs, and put her outside with Kundun. When they both come back into the house, I realize that Tara has never come downstairs. I go back upstairs and she is still on the bed in Rasa's place. She won't get off the bed. By now I'm becoming irritated. It's too early. I haven't had my tea. I go back downstairs and grab Tara's leash, go back upstairs and loop it around her neck. I am brusque about getting her off the bed. She seems reluctant to move. So, I say, "Come on. Come on." Finally she jumps off the bed, but I don't watch her jump off the bed. When I look back at her while she is on the wood floor going around a corner, I see her hind legs slipping and whirling. When I think back about this, I have no idea how she jumped off the bed or got down the tile stairs to the kitchen at all.

Tara won't go outside to pee. She goes in to the medium size crate which sits next to Kundun's large size crate. I feed her in the crate and she eats lightly while lying down then curls up and doesn't move. I shower, dress, and go back to the kitchen. I look in the crate and see that she has peed and is lying in it, the cushion completely soggy and wet. I pull the bed out of the crate with her on it. She staggers six feet to her Orvis green plaid bagel bed and collapses. As I gently stroke Tara on her head and back, I talk to her softly as a surge of panic rises up inside me. Somehow I get a potty pad under her without one growl.

I feel heartless, stupid, impatient and utterly overwhelmed. I call Buena Animal Hospital, "Tara has an emergency and I need to bring her in immediately."

A man who helps me with little handyman type projects comes to the house. We pick up the bed with Tara in it, a terrified look on her face, carry her out of the kitchen and heft her into the back of my SUV. At Buena she is carried in bed and all. They disappear into the back and I sit in the waiting room scared for my beloved Tara.

After what seems like hours, Dr. Nicci comes into the waiting room and sits down next to me. She looks really serious, so I dread the prognosis.

"She has a fibro-cartilaginous embolism."

I have no idea what this means except for the word embolism, and can only say, "Oh shit." I slap my hand over my mouth, "I'm sorry. What is it?"

"The cause is unknown, but what happens is that a tiny piece of cartilage breaks off and floats in the spinal fluid. It then blocks the fluid like a blood clot blocking an artery. The result is a paralysis of the hind end."

I immediately think of the dog that lived in a house next to the Animal Clinic parking lot in Santa Fe. The dog couldn't use its hind end, so the owner had rigged up a little two wheel cart to strap the dog's hind quarters into. The dog ran around the yard with its cart, and I was always amazed at how normal the dog acted.

"Tara will have to stay here for five days. I have to give her steroid injections, keep her on IVs, and monitor her progress."

I sign the paperwork, pay the deposit, and take her empty bed to the car. I drive home eyes blurred with tears. My whole world is crashing down, and I feel absolutely, completely lost in this ocean of critical dog illnesses. The following day I take in Tara's food and supplements plus her favorite purple fuzzy dolly. I do a few errands in Ojai, absentmindedly pick up cleaning, purchase a few groceries then drive home on Creek Road. I wail, "Not Tara! Please, not Tara!" I yell and cry in my car. I can't do it at home—it will upset Rasa and Kundun. After the nightmare of moving, the stress of workmen around endlessly, trying to figure out how to hike with hounds on leashes—now they are physically collapsing before my eyes.

Five days later I arrive at Buena to pick up Tara. When I see her I gasp in horror. All of her vertebrae protrude. Her defined back muscles are gone. Her belly is swollen. Her back looks swayed. This is from the steroids. My hardy, fit, muscular, beautiful girl looks like a pot-bellied pig. She has a sling with handles around her belly. The vet techs show me how to hold the handles to lift most of her weight off her feet to walk and to get her in and out of the car.

Dr. Nicci warns me, "She is fragile. She cannot run and has to be confined. She must stay on flat surfaces and has to be leash-walked to pee and poop."

Tara goes up and down the stairs seemingly completely cured. However, I am being lenient, happy to have her home. She collapses and has to be rushed to the clinic again. She stays for two days. When I pick her up Dr. Nicci makes it very clear that Tara must be confined to one room, no stairs, no excitement. When she walks she has to use the canvas sling.

Tara stays in the kitchen. With the threat of permanent damage and the miracle of complete recovery, I now supervise every moment of her day. The kitchen is a large room with glass doors and windows that look out into a river rock paved courtyard shaded by large live oaks, and up the grass covered hill above the house. A fountain that sounds like a small creek is against the wall across from the glass doors. Tara's bed is at the end of the dining table in front of a glass door. She can lie in her bed and keep her eye on the hillside for anything of interest. In this way she has spotted a raccoon, coyotes frequently, a great blue heron and two deer. Of course spotting them is only the beginning. Then she barks, goes to the door and wants out. Before the embolism, Rasa and Tara would charge out the door and up the hill to the fence around their yard. They ran up and down the fence barking long after whatever it was had run into the bushes to hide, or flown away. I learned quickly after we moved here to go out with the dogs to see what they are barking at as they wildly run back and forth along their fence. Rasa and Tara think that the heron is a wild turkey. How they loved to chase wild turkeys in New Mexico. The turkeys would run faster and faster then take off into the air. The dogs could never figure out what happened to them, where they went, so they would run in circles with noses to the ground, Tara baying. The deer were a huge surprise, and by the time I saw them the dogs were out the door and the deer were bounding up the hill.

I sit in my armed dining chair at the other end of the table from Tara's bed to drink tea, read magazines or books, and write. I sit here in the late afternoons to have a snack, to eat dinner a little later and to watch the news on T.V. There is Kundun's large rattan crate in the opposite corner. The door is left open, and inside the crate is a heated bio-pad filled with amethyst crystals which is turned on all of the time. Next to that is a smaller rattan crate, and near my chair is another dog bed. So, this is our family gathering place. There is the favorite bed for each dog, the second choice bed for two dogs, and the never used bed by Tara in the crate. A little room off the kitchen that I call the butler's pantry has a third, even smaller rattan crate tucked under the counter where a chair may have been placed by a previous owner. I put this crate there for Tara, because she becomes so fearful that I think she needs a hiding place.

On one particularly bad morning after Pecos has returned home, he completely trashes the laundry room. I clean that up, and I clean up the kitchen from Tara, because the steroids cause her to pee all night as they did Rasa. My energy is non-existent, my buttons are all pushed to the extreme—I lose it and start yelling. I go upstairs to shower and dress. When I return downstairs I try to make amends, to calm down. Kundun is hunkered down in his crate looking at me with big brown fearful eyes. I can't find Tara. Finally I locate her curled up in the small crate in the butler's pantry facing the back of it and completely unwilling to move. I pet and stroke her, apologize, and keep going back, but she is unmoved by me. Feeling like a self-destructing monster, I sit in my chair and begin to cry. I cannot stop. All of the frustration, fear of losing my dogs, the unbelievable ordeal of moving, my helplessness in the face of ongoing critical animal care becomes a river of tears. I absolutely cannot act like this for one more minute of my life. I am scaring the dogs. I am scaring myself.

When Tara finally emerges she has streams of teary gunk coming out of her eyes. We are both crying.

5

realize that Pecos has to go back to Cindy's and stay there long term. Cindy's Cat Vacations is in a derelict, boarded up, mostly vacant looking area called Wagon Wheel. There is a hotel in disrepair and abandoned. The kennel itself is a solitary building surrounded by a high chain link fence with a locked gate. The first time I arrived with Pecos, I almost had a heart attack when I saw the neighborhood and kennel building, believing I had made a serious mistake. However, as I waited with my car doors locked parked on the street in front of the fence, Cindy arrived in her mini-van, unlocked the gate and drove in. I followed her in the door to a comfy office with an overstuffed chair and all things cats. She opened up a garage type door to let the sun and a breeze come in through the wood latticework across the opening. Cats of every size and color were everywhere together in a big room. My fears subsided and I knew that Pecos would like it here, plus Cindy loves cats and intensely takes care of them as if each one is her own.

Cindy, a plump, middle-age, motherly person explains, "This area has been purchased by a developer to build two condominium towers, but with the economy, nothing has happened yet. I rent month to month. The Wagon Wheel Hotel used to be a popular, fancy place where many Hollywood stars would spend the weekend in the nineteen-thirties."

"I don't know how long Pecos will be here. He is very difficult to feed. He likes fish, especially salmon, eats some kibble, drinks a lot of water and sleeps. He likes to be part of a group—the pride, the pack, so as long as he can hang out with all of the other cats he is happy even if he's asleep."

After I return home, I feel a huge relief, and I have a glimpse of just why it is that people end up in nursing homes. I clean up everything that belongs to Pecos and put the cat box in the garage. His beds sit empty—one in the kitchen and one in the laundry room. His special little dishes are stacked up on the shelf.

Next I begin to monitor my moods and my mouth. Once I start to think about it, I realize that I have suffered depression for years, beginning in New Mexico. I lived in an isolated, rugged area east of Pecos. I lived alone. Because of the seventy mile round trip drive to Santa Fe, I had eliminated a lot of my social life. I found that driving at night was a challenge as I would get confused. Driving at night in inclement weather was dangerous. The last three miles home were two miles of a poorly maintained dirt road, and one mile of completely unmaintained dirt four-wheel-drive road that was bedrock in some places. I would try to meet friends early for dinner to eliminate dark drives. I was relegated to week nights because they were busy with boyfriends on weekends, and early didn't seem to work for any but one friend, who in the process became best friend and only friend.

Because of the forty-five minute drive one way, I planned way ahead for these dinners. The dogs would be fed early, go out to run around, then come indoors while I was gone. I became annoyed to listen to a complaint about the need to rush home from yoga to shower and meet me so early, or someone else rousing herself from a nap to meet me thirty minutes late after I had ordered and eaten. So, the dinner dates diminished as did the phone calls and I became more isolated.

I tried to hire caretakers to live in the apartment that I built over the garage, but ended up firing every one and having none the last two years that I lived there. I had one man who tried to kill my horses by hiding gravel in the grain. This would have caused colic or intestinal blockage. Fortunately I found the rocks as I poured the grain from the scoop into the stall feeder on a weekend when he was gone. I dug through the can finding more and more. He was fired immediately. Another man had a sarcastic way of talking to me. He tried to steal everything on the way out, and he wouldn't leave. He had the keys to every door on the place and my dogs knew him. I had called the sheriff's office for a back-up, and followed their advice with a written notice. If he did not leave they would escort him off the property. I had been holed up in my house for two weeks, had run out of food, and was afraid to leave because he might come in and steal things. Finally at the appointed moment to pick up the phone and call the sheriff, he drove out. I had all of the locks changed the next day.

Finally, years later, a few days before my birthday, I broke two of my own rules. I didn't cancel dinner with a friend when I saw snowflakes beginning to fall just as it was time to leave on the drive into Santa Fe, and I had agreed to go to a music concert after dinner. Everything seemed fine after the concert, no snow. I headed home on I-25, and as I turned the big curve just past the Lamy exit there was a blinding curtain of snow with accumulated snow on the ground. I slowed down but not enough, and I did not shift into 4WD. The pavement looked black and wet. Small cars were passing me, so I couldn't tell if it was ice or not. My speed was approximately 50mph. Suddenly I fish-tailed and was headed toward the median strip and oncoming south bound traffic. I knew that whatever I did would cause a big problem, but hitting other cars head-on was not an option. I barely turned the steering wheel without using the brakes. This sent me fish-tailing the opposite direction toward the right shoulder of the north bound lane. At the place I left the road there was no guardrail, or I would have bounced off that and probably hit cars behind me who could not brake without doing what I was doing.

My Toyota 4-Runner quietly rolled completely over and when it was back on its wheels began to move forward. I slammed my foot on the brake, threw it in park, hit the emergency flashers, and looked at the inside of the car. The passenger window was gone, as was everything on the passenger seat including my purse. A man and woman arrived at my window.

"You've got a flat tire," he offered.

I found this enormously funny given that I had just rolled and probably totaled my SUV.

"Call 911," she ordered.

"You call 911, I'm calling my son."

"Turn the engine off."

"No, it's too cold. Can you please look for my purse back there—it must have fallen out of the window when it broke."

The man returned with my purse, wallet, which had fallen out of the purse, paper bag with my birthday gift in it, hat, and assorted other things that flew out. It was eerily quiet in the snow. I was way below the road, so I couldn't see anything. I thanked them for helping me, and began to stuff everything in my purse from the console.

My son arrived as they were loading me into the ambulance, "It wasn't hard to find you—there are flashing lights on both sides of the freeway."

I, of course, had expected to get in his car and go home. The EMT's gave me a scary dialogue about broken necks and severed spinal cords. So, I spent hours in the emergency room of St. Vincent's Hospital in Santa Fe. The fact that everyone in Santa Fe called it St. Victims did not make me excited to be there. I wouldn't let them cut off my new wool coat with fur trim. After determining that I didn't have any internal injuries or a broken neck, they finally they let me go.

I returned home at two in the morning, the lights on, dogs eager to see me. My son immediately left to return to Santa Fe as the snow was piling up, and he was concerned about getting out with worn down tires. I sat at home for several days contemplating how I could have been killed so easily in that accident. This was my turning point. I couldn't live in this rugged isolation any longer. It was time to ramp up the search for a home in California, and move before the next winter. If I didn't move before winter, the moving truck wouldn't be able to get in to move me out. This gave me nine months to enjoy my last summer and autumn in my beloved valley, to take my last hikes on my trails, to say goodbye to every little detail after twenty years.

6

aura arrives for our appointment. Rasa, Tara, and Kundun are excited to see her and she is happy to see them. We gather in the kitchen. I sit in my customary armchair at the end of the table, Laura sits in the other armchair which is on the side of the table, and the dogs all lie on the beds that are not in crates.

"What do you want to ask them today?"

I recall a walk that Rasa and Tara and I took on a long sandy beach near Ventura Harbor before the cancer, before the embolism when my girls seemed so healthy and strong. Tara had never seen the ocean before we moved here, and when we would walk on the beach she completely avoided the water moving up and down the sand. However, on this day she started walking in the shallow waves and facing the ocean. All I could see were sailboats far out in the water. We continued our walk to a place where Snowy Plovers were nesting. The birds made a whistle sound similar to a New Mexico ground squirrel. Oh, happy hunting! Rasa started digging holes in the sand. She would cock her head sideways, listen, then start digging another hole. This was very funny to me and when I kept pointing to the birds overhead, a man sitting there watched us very amused.

On the way back Tara headed right into the water, the waves, and if I wouldn't have had her on a leash, I think she would have started swimming straight out. I looked and looked.

"What do you smell or see Tara? Oh wow, a pod of dolphins!" They were way out there so I was curious about how she knew that.

"Ask Tara how she knew about the dolphins, and tell her that they are dolphins."

Tara and Laura have a long conversation. "Tara could hear them."

"Dolphins are hawks of the water—playful and graceful. I want to be a dolphin when I come back."

"Wait, how do you know about reincarnation?" Laura asks.

"I killed a rat, and I saw its spirit leave."

"Oh, Tara is the one who killed the rat."

This was when my house in New Mexico was over-run with rodents after Pecos retired. I was leaving to have dinner in Santa Fe with my family and a rat ran out from under the sofa. Rasa jumped off her bed three feet away and grabbed it in her mouth then dropped it. I put on my rubber gloves, got a plastic bag and bent down to pick it up by the tail. It jumped and ran back under the sofa. I screamed. On my way out the door I instructed to anyone listening, "Kill that god-damned thing!" When I returned home from dinner there was the rat, dead, lying in Tara's bed. I praised everyone.

"Ask Rasa why she eats dirt and poop?"

"Dirt makes me feel more alert. I eat poop because I'm hungry."

"There is simply no way to feed Rasa as much food as she thinks she needs, because the prednisone is giving her a voracious appetite. I have tried every anti-poop eating product there is, and nothing works. I try to clean up the dog yard more frequently, and I watch her, then yell a stern 'Leave it!' from the door. Hopefully when the time comes to go off the prednisone, this behavior will end."

Rasa randomly interjects, "Kundun has to drink his dinner."

Laura looks baffled, and talks to Kundun, "My food at the kennel is full of water."

Rasa wasn't at the kennel when Tara and Kundun last stayed there, so I immediately realize that my dogs are communicating with each other from a distance. This is one of the two times Rasa accompanied me to L.A. I take all of my dogs' food to the kennel for them with written instructions, so the liquid meals don't sound good.

"There are dogs at the kennel that don't have homes."

Kundun is very upset by this, and indeed the kennel is a rescue sanctuary that also boards dogs to bring in income. I realize that this is not an ideal situation for Kundun. More than that I am reminded of how Kundun came into my life, homeless and scared. Now having a home is all he knows, and he treasures that.

Late on a day in early January I was driving home in my pick-up truck. The sun had set behind me dropping below Rowe Mesa and it was becoming dark. A storm had moved in from the west and snowflakes were drifting down.

Ahead of me coming the opposite direction was a blue pick-up truck that slowed down and stopped on the side of the road. I in turn slowed down and watched it. Vehicles that did stop in this area always parked in a certain location on the other side of a cattle guard at the end of the paved road before it divided into two dirt roads. This was different. I saw the driver get out of the truck. He went around to the back. At this point I was even with the truck and could not see what he was doing. He walked back, got in his truck and drove away. By now I was crawling along and looking in my rearview mirror. That's when I saw a puppy chasing behind the truck. I thought, what a stupid way to exercise a dog, then I realized that they had dumped him! The truck speeded off and there was the puppy all alone on the side of the road. I backed up, parked and tried to catch the puppy, but he ran into a culvert under the road. I had on a skirt and boots for town, so I went home to change clothes, grab some dog treats, and get back three miles to try to rescue a dog that would surely not make it through the night with the cold, coyotes, bobcats, and occasional mountain lion in the area. As soon as I got to my gate, I saw a small herd of cows standing by the fence that crosses the Ojo Sarco Creek where it exits my land to flow down the valley. I had no choice but to open the gate, get the truck out of the way, and with skirt and knee-high boots clamber through the snow yelling to chase them out.

It was almost dark now. I drove to the house, unloaded the groceries, changed clothes, grabbed some dog biscuits, and my neighbor. We drove back to the culvert and there was the puppy. I had Wesley stand at the opposite end of the culvert and I held out the treat and called. He ran up to get the food, snatched it out of my hand and kept going. I tackled him, scooped him up, and plopped him in the back of my red Toyota Tundra with a camper shell. By the time I arrived home it was completely dark, snowing heavily, and the thermometer on the front porch registered zero. I retrieved the crate Rasa and Tara had arrived in from Georgia over one year before, and moved it from the garage to the house. The only place left to put anything in my jam-packed small log house was next to my bedroom door. I fed him and he was famished - his ribs stuck out. He arrived with huge over-size ears, big white paws, a broad white chest with the rest of him a beautiful brindle color, and looked like a pit bull mix with the tiniest white triangle on his nose.

I didn't have the heart to take him to the shelter in Santa Fe. Their policy is to immediately euthanize all pit bulls. The animal sanctuary nearby in Glorieta wouldn't take a pit bull. I took him for vaccinations to Dr. Hinko at the Animal Clinic in Santa Fe, "He's three to four months old." That put his birthday in approximately September, a Virgo. He would fit right in with the Catahoula Leos. I named him Kundun and it fit him perfectly.

Kundun followed me everywhere. I would stop to turn around to look for him and he would run into the back of my leg. He gained weight, became less frightened, and every night when I tucked him into his crate, I would tell him, "You did everything right today, Kundun. You did everything right." He had been so abused, and yet all he wanted to do was to please me. I never had to train him. He learned everything by observing the other dogs and figuring it out himself. Kabuki, my aging Akita, could not be bothered with puppies, but he would let Kundun curl up next to him without the obligatory growl and move to another location. Kabuki had to be euthanized seven months later, but I never lost him. Kabuki's quirky personality lives on in Kundun, as does his ear to ear grin. After trying to find a home for Kundun for six months I realized that I was too attached to him to let him go. By now he has huge ears that stand up like radars and a long tail that never stops wagging. It thumps in his crate, bangs against kitchen cupboards, and rotates in a circle behind him like a helicopter propeller when he runs. He tucks his ears back when he is being friendly. His eyes are the deepest, darkest brown and watch everything.

Laura talks again to Kundun.

"I want to make new friends and play with them." This from the pit bull that had a job at the ranch—chase away neighbor dogs, feral dogs, and look fierce to anyone driving in who wasn't expected. Kundun has a gentle manner about him, but when he is in watch dog mode he is absolutely frightening. He pushes his chest out and reveals super-size gleaming white teeth as he rushes forward growling and barking in a deep voice.

Tara has been quietly lying in her bed, "When I couldn't walk we both cried. The birds stopped singing. When I got well, the birds began to sing again."

Laura and I look at each other wordlessly as Tara's profound poetry fills the space around us. I think of that morning and everything the tears imply. I silently remind myself that it will never happen again. I am going to practice
• loving kindness until it is who I am no matter what is happening that pushes
• my flip-out button.

We end our session at the end of an hour and say goodbye.

7

Thanksgiving and Christmas come and go. Rasa's ten weeks of chemo end along with the Wednesday commute to Woodland Hills. Tara recovers enough to get in and out of the side door of the SUV, and to go up and down the stairs plus jump on the bed. Sometimes I hear a crash and run to the stairs to find her spread-eagled on the tile steps. I help her up. I place a carpet scrap on the landing which helps. It seems to be that partial corner that causes the largest problem maneuvering the stairs. Sometimes her back legs tremble and shake uncontrollably at night. I hold on to her legs until it stops.

Kundun begins to go to a new kennel where the dogs intermingle during the day and employees play with the dogs in a large fenced area with trees. He seems very happy going there and they love him. When I leave Tara there as well, after her embolism, I am very worried. I leave the food, the written feeding instructions, and a special letter about Tara's physical issues and request that she not be placed in with other dogs. Of course, my wishes are completely ignored and when I arrive to pick them up I am horrified to see Tara in with the other dogs. She is standing off by herself looking uncomfortable with the situation.

In early February Laura arrives for a conversation.

"Kundun's arthritis is becoming increasingly worse," I explain.

"A secret medicine from deep in the earth would make the pain go away," Kundun states.

Laura and I look at each other helplessly not knowing what this could possibly be.

"My life feels like lots of flowers. The cancer is gone, I don't need any more chemo," Rasa announces.

Rasa goes once a month for chemotherapy now. She still takes the chemo capsules orally every other day, the pepsid, the prednisone. The prednisone makes her grumpy. She growls at Kundun and Tara. She shreds her dolls. Sometimes she even growls at me.

"Can we communicate with Bhakti in New Mexico? He is my son's Weimaraner."

"I need a photograph of him."

"Oh dear, I haven't found those yet in the process of unpacking. He looks like one of William Wegman's classic photos of Weimaraners on the greeting cards."

I don't understand how it works, but Laura locates Bhakti. He is older than my dogs, by now twelve. He has beautiful light amber eyes, is a dusty gray color, and is a bouncy, loopy big dog with a loving heart.

Laura looks puzzled, "Does he eat barbeque? He says he wants a barbeque."

My daughter is visiting and has joined us with her English Mastiff, Crush. "We had family barbeques in Pecos at either Mom's ranch or mine. The family would all be there and all of the dogs. We would all hike together then cook dinner on the grill. That's what he means."

Poor Bhakti, he misses his extended family of people and dogs, and the years of barbeques since he was a puppy. "Tell him we all miss him."

"I want to be with people who love me when I die."

"Tell him Kabuki and Wuli will be waiting for him."

"They are all with me now."

I feel sad when we "hang up."

Laura begins to engage Crush. She is ready to give up trying to converse with him when he finally seems to understand how it works. Crush is huge and he is slow. Cassidy wants to know if he thinks anything has worked in his regimen of dealing with skin issues, allergies, and fungus.

"Two times ago when I went to the vet."

"Crush's vet spends a lot of time thinking about Crush's problems, and how to fix them," Rasa states.

Tara ends the session, "I'm afraid of coyotes at night."

Laura recommends that we go see Cynthia, a nutritionist, who works with dogs and people. I make an appointment.

Cassidy calls, "Antibiotics."

"What are you talking about?"

"Two times ago Crush's vet prescribed antibiotics. He's back on them now and probably will be for the rest of his life."

Again I'm amazed at the wisdom of the dogs, and how much information is in their minds that we don't realize. I'm taken with how they communicate and how their individual personalities emerge beyond what I ever could have guessed.

Pecos has now been at Cindy's for three months. I think things have settled down enough with the dogs to bring him home. I decide to do that at the end of the month. I recall the dream I had after I left him the second time. Pecos sits very still in the sun next to a barn door. Wuli stands further away from the barn, dark brown eyes watching him.

Cassidy and Crush arrive for the weekend to celebrate my birthday. On Saturday evening we enjoy my birthday dinner at Azu's in Ojai. We are joined by friends and it is a wonderful celebration with lots of laughter. We all say goodbye with many hugs and kisses, then Cassidy and I drive home. The phone rings. I look at the clock. It is ten P.M. I hesitantly pick up the phone from the kitchen table.

It is Cindy. She is crying, "Something has happened to Pecos. I think he's had a stroke. I'm not sure he'll make it to the morning."

I confer with Cassidy. She will drive me there immediately. I don't want to drive at night. "I'll be there in thirty minutes. Are you at the kennel?"

We change clothes and head for Oxnard. When we arrive, we walk in the unlocked door. Cindy is sitting in the over-stuffed chair with Pecos wrapped in a blue cotton baby blanket curled up in a basket with a handle, which she is holding in her lap. He looks very fragile, thin and old since I have last seen him. Cindy has tears in her eyes. I lean down and touch Pecos' head. "Hello Pecos. I'm here." He emits a weak squeaky meow in response.

Cindy stands up, motions for me to sit down and hands me the basket with Pecos. A few minutes pass, and Cassidy asks, "What do you want to do?"

"We'll take him home now."

Since I sleep with Rasa and Tara on the bed and they take up over one-half of a California king size bed, Cassidy offers to have Pecos sleep with her in the guest room. I move him to his round fleece bed leaving him in the little blue blanket. It appears that his hind end is paralyzed, and that he cannot see. He spends the night in his bed on top of the guest bed with my daughter's hand touching him all night.

In the morning I move him from the guest room to the kitchen where I place his bed in the dining armchair facing and next to my chair. Rasa keeps sticking her nose in to check on him. He is near my chair so I can touch him. I think because he can't see, he keeps making little squeaky meows to get a response so that he knows where I am. Pecos refuses to take any water which I am attempting to give him with an eyedropper. He doesn't pee, he doesn't drink. He is thin and weak.

Here I am with Pecos at the end of his eighteen and one-half year life. One paw sticks out of the top of the bed. Rasa sticks her nose close and jumps back. I see blood, and think Pecos got one last swipe at her. On closer inspection I see that Rasa's entire face is covered with nasty looking bumps and that Pecos' claw protruding from his immobile paw ripped open one of these when Rasa's head came close to it. Because Rasa's face is black, white and blue spotted, and even with glasses I miss details, I have not noticed this. I make a mental note to call the vet in the morning about the bumps.

I take Kundun with me to look for a place to bury Pecos uphill from the oak grove. After his cat friend, Cimarron, died Pecos was afraid to go outside alone. He knew that he couldn't climb trees or run anymore. I discovered that he would go out if Kundun was with him, so a special relationship developed. Kundun had learned the art of a slow, quiet tip-toe up to a pocket gopher hole and poising soundlessly with one paw raised looking like a bulky bird dog until the gopher moved out to eat grass. Then he would pounce like a cat and grab it. He learned this from Kabuki. For Kundun the game was in the hunting and catching then he would drop the gopher on the ground. It didn't take Pecos long to figure out that a delicious meal awaited him at the end of this, and I would find body parts on the porch.

I find a place beneath a pepper tree. There is shade. There is sun. It looks down at the house from the hillside. The hole is dug. When it is time to go to bed, I move Pecos, bed and all to the laundry room and place his bed where it always was since our move on the bottom shelf of a large open storage cupboard. I turn on the heater. I stroke his head, feel his ears yellow and soft between my fingers.

"Good night Pecos. I love you. I'm sorry about all of the times I ever got angry about the cat box. I know you couldn't help it. You've been a good kitty. Say hello to Cimarron and Calico—they'll be happy to see you. Bye, bye little buddy." I turn out the light and close the door.

In the morning he is gone, his paw frozen sticking up to the top of the bed. And that is how I met him—sticking his paw out of the cage at the shelter to grab my shoulder, "Take me!" Now it is a silent farewell. He is stiff, and I think maybe he left the moment I closed that door. I move him out of his bed and discover that his other front foot is bent uncomfortably, claws caught in the fabric of the blanket. I feel badly about not noticing this before. I wrap him in the blue blanket and wrap a towel with a leopard pattern around that. I choose a glass heart from my heart collection and place it in his grave with him. Like every other cat and dog I've buried I face his head toward the east, shovel in the dirt, pile up rocks to keep the coyotes out, and sprinkle rose petals on top. It begins to rain as soon as I am finished. An extra blessing.

I remember the article that a Buddhist lama wrote. He postulated that we shouldn't euthanize our pets. It was his belief that we Americans do it as a matter of convenience. I had euthanized several aging and infirm dogs over the years. Each was done by the local Pecos vet who came out to my ranch. Each dog was in my lap no matter how large. Each dog had a ceremony done by a Native American friend. Each death brought tears and an empty feeling in my home. I thought I had done the right thing. I had wrestled with the thought of having Pecos euthanized and buried next to his buddy, Cimarron, on the land he had known all his life. In fact I struggled with this for three years as his condition worsened. But the lama's words haunted me and I didn't do that. There is a deep resonance in this moment, this event happening on its own volition that allows me to let go without remorse. I am sad, but I am relieved for both of us.

Dr. Nicci cannot figure out what is causing Rasa's bumps. She puts her on an antibiotic concluding that with the chemo and prednisone her immune system is down, and that this could be from sticking her nose in the dirt and picking up some normally insignificant bacteria.

I board Rasa at the vet when Kundun and Tara are at the kennel because her rabies is not current, she should not have a rabies vaccination while on chemo, and she is on so much medication that a vet tech needs to deal with it. I leave for a ten day trip north to visit my sister in Napa. When I get Rasa back home I see that not only did the antibiotics not cure the bumps, they have spread all over her body. I am irritated—she was at the vet for ten days. Is anyone paying attention? I take her back and the antibiotic is changed, plus I am advised to have her bathed with a special shampoo.

Finally this problem clears up however every bump has left a small patch of black hair where it was white before, so her face looks different now. It looks moth-eaten or still bumpy without the bumps. Of course she doesn't know this.

8

When I call Cynthia to make our appointment, she says, "I can have two dogs come." I make a tough choice and arrive with Rasa and Kundun. What I don't realize is that she is treating my dogs and me.

Cynthia looks at all of us from behind her desk. We are upstairs in her office, which is in her Victorian house overlooking the Ventura River valley to the west. Cynthia is prim with a twinkle in her eyes. "Tell me everyone's symptoms."

I start with myself. "I can't sleep. I'm a nervous wreck, tired all of the time, crabby. I can't seem to accomplish more than caring for dogs and getting through my day, plus I've recently realized that I've been in a state of depression for years before I moved to California, and I'm still struggling with that.

"Kundun has arthritis that is increasingly worse and nothing the vet prescribes seems to help. He is becoming more and more immobile. Rasa is on chemotherapy, prednisone, a million supplements, and hopefully recovering from her mast cell skin cancer in the process."

Cynthia smiles, "Do you know the kind of work that I do?"

"No, I don't know anything." I instantly suspect that this is going to be more than nutrition.

"I use a process that is based on the theory that your body will heal itself if it is told what to do. This process is called sound balancing. You hold this little vial, and tuck this in Kundun's collar, and this one in Rasa's collar. Then I play a recording of a tuning fork based on sacred geometry. Do you know what sacred geometry is?"

"Yes, I know that it is based on the mathematical equations that occur naturally in nature, such as the ripples formed when you throw a stone into a pool of water, and how far apart those ripples are, which is always the same."

I tuck the vials into Rasa's and Kundun's collars. They are pacing and roving around nervously. The second the mesmerizing "music" begins, they each lie down and remain still. Meanwhile, Cynthia is opening black boxes of rows of vials which are stacked on her desk and open like binders. She touches different bottles with her little finger while she muscle tests each of us by pushing on her thumb while her hand is facing toward whoever she is testing. It is all very mysterious.

"Well, first we work on toxins to get them out of the body; pesticides, and DDT. That will reveal other issues. I want you to start feeding them raw food. I've had dogs completely cured of arthritis by going off dry food and eating a raw diet."

We make an appointment for the next week. Rasa and Kundun get a treat and home we go. I explore our local organic pet store, Noah's Apothecary, to find raw food. It is expensive. I decide that I can feed three dogs raw food once a day and they will have to stay on dry, although half as much dry. The complete raw diet with ground hearts, livers and bones is more expensive than the ground chicken or turkey with vegetables which necessitates feeding dry for a complete diet. I am not certain that I will accomplish much with a partial raw diet, but I decide to give it a try.

Rasa, Kundun and I visit Cynthia weekly for several weeks. Our bodies all continue to eliminate toxins from the environment.

Cynthia describes her work this way, "I use 'testing vials' in conjunction with the sound healing in an attempt to assess how the client is responding to the work. These are vials of water with energy imprints in them. Based on the information from the vials and client feedback, the sound healing system appears to accomplish several things. First, the 'sound balances,' as I call the sessions seem to activate detoxification within the body, getting it to release chemicals, heavy metals, old pharmaceutical residues and the like. This clean-up throughout the body in turn appears to result in improved absorption of nutrients, as toxicity is widely believed to obstruct nutritional absorption. As the body becomes cleaner and better nourished, many common problems improve including allergies, low energy, poor immune function, poor sleep, hormonal and mood fluctuations, and some pain syndromes.

"Second, the sound balances appear to activate the immune system to better address pathogens such as bacteria, viruses, parasites and funguses like candida. As the immune system becomes more capable, problems such as chronic colds and flus, digestive complaints associated with parasites and a wide range of problems associated with candida such as brain fog, poor sleep, irritability, mood and hormonal fluctuations, fatigue, food cravings, etc. can improve.

"Overall, for clients who are strong enough to tolerate the detoxification process, the sound balancing work can result in improved feelings of well-being, including more energy, mental clarity and mood stability, and fewer episodes of common illnesses, allergic reactivity and digestive complaints."

2

Kundun goes into the oak grove on the land next door before going to bed. He likes to wander around sniffing and marking. The land has a gentle slope, so it is easier for him to walk. Tonight, however, as the sky begins to darken, Kundun melts into the shadows, his brindle color invisible against the background. I call, but he doesn't come like usual. I call and call becoming irritated that he is ignoring me. I worry because of the coyotes. When I moved here I was told the same dire story repeatedly—one coyote will lure your dog and the rest of the pack will wait at a distance to kill it. In New Mexico we lived where there were coyotes, bears, and mountain lions. I never worried about the dogs. But now my dogs are older only they don't know it. Once it is completely dark I start to panic, and I get more upset. Kundun has never come to an angry sounding voice, so I am trying to sound calm, happy, and upbeat while I am ready to kill him if the coyotes don't.

During our session following that situation I say to Laura, "Tell Kundun that I wasn't mad at him when he disappeared and wouldn't come when I called him. I was worried about him."

"I knew you weren't mad at me. I was upset that you were upset. Now I'm acting and being perfect. I went out at night to show you I'm not afraid. I talked to an owl. The owl said that she likes watching our family. I asked her what she eats. She said snakes and rabbits. I told her I'd like to eat a rabbit. She said she wouldn't share a rabbit with me. Cynthia thinks I am perfect. She makes my head more clear. My toes, neck, and back hurt—most in the morning. Tara feels left out not going to Cynthia and that makes me sad."

"The trees love it when I run through them!" Rasa exclaims.

Tara has a much different experience in the oak grove next door, "I'm scared to go out without Mom. I have anxiety and can't breathe. I can't think when I can't breathe. The shadows scare me."

Recently when Cassidy was visiting we all went out into the oak grove. Tara immediately disappeared into the center of the grove and didn't come when

I called her. Cassidy waded down the slope covered with years of accumulated fallen, dead, sharp-edged oak leaves and found Tara standing there. "She's right here, call her."

Tara emerged from the dark into the lights in the driveway. It is very clear that I need to take her on a leash from now on when we go out for the final potty break at night. We go next door because there are lights on the garage and we can see. Also there are no steps or a steep hill to maneuver. It is a grove of huge old live oaks, home to squirrels and many species of birds hunting for the bounty of acorns scattered beneath them. It is where the coyote trail crosses before rising up the hill above our house. Even with a full moon it is dark below the canopy of branches.

Tara adds one more comment, "Sometimes I don't know who someone is even when I do, until the other dogs recognize them. When there are too many people in the house, the energy is confusing to me."

I believe that Tara is losing her eyesight, but perhaps it is more than that because she certainly doesn't miss the coyotes on the hill above the house. However, Tara could smell them before she sees them. Frequently she sniffs at the crack between the opening and fixed halves of the glass door going from the kitchen to the courtyard. In any case, Tara has a fragile mental state and I am very protective of her for that reason. She does bark at everyone in the house even if they just spent the night upstairs in the guestroom. I give her Rescue Remedy every morning.

"Tell Rasa she is on Dr. Alice's cure list!"

"I'm so excited to be on the cure list! If Kundun is perfect—I am even better. We only talk to Laura if we have problems, and I feel perfect! I want to go into town. I want to go somewhere fun. Tara needs to go to Cynthia to become perfect so she can catch up with us."

Rasa's attitude is infectious, and I know that we've been home way too much with excursions limited to trips to the vet endlessly for the past year. The chemotherapy has been hard on Rasa. She looks older now. The prednisone has made her grumpy and aggressive toward Kundun and Tara. It has given her a voracious appetite. To try to keep her from eating poop, I feed her more, but the inactivity has allowed her to gain weight. When the coyotes come, I let the dogs out to bark and run back and forth along the fence, because it's the best exercise she gets.

We are a family, a pack, and I'm very taken by the concern Rasa and Kundun have for Tara being left out and needing to catch up with them in the healing process at Cynthia's. At our next appointment I explain this to her.

"Well, I'm certain it will work to have all three dogs here. Bring her."

10

While I am enveloped in dog health drama, I spend less and less time with my beloved Paso Fino gelding. Genji is fourteen now. When I bought him he was a handsome dappled dun three year old stallion with black legs from his knees to his hooves, a black mane and tail plus a dorsal stripe from his withers to his tail. I rode many horses at the stable in Florida where he was for sale, but Genji won my heart with his elegant color, dark eyes, and what in the Paso Fino breed is called *brio*. Brio is best defined as an attitude, a state of mind, a heart for the joy of the ride. This kind of Paso Fino is described as *con mucho brio*.

BRIO

Jorge, the owner of the stable with his wife, told me, "He just came in this morning. I could sell him for twice as much, but you are here today, and I'll give you a good price." I didn't bargain with his price it was so fair. I had my new horse gelded, and named him Genji after my most favorite character in a Japanese book titled, "A Tale of Genji." This book was actually the first novel ever written, and by a woman, Lady Murasaki, a member of the royal court in Heian Japan in approximately the year 1000 A.C.E. Genji means shining, but not like light reflecting off a surface, which is called *hikari*—it is a brilliance of beauty and other-worldly perfection.

The Paso Fino breed is descended from the Barb horse, a North African Barbary Coast breed that dates back over two thousand years to Libyan tribes that kept the breed pure for centuries. They are not to be confused with Arabian horses. The Barb is known for its agility and high stepping action adapted to the rocky, rough mountainous desert. The Moors crossed their Barbs with the remnants of the Andalusian breed. One of the main genetic lines to develop was the now extinct Spanish Jennet with a smooth gait and the ability to pass this along to its offspring.

A different type of horse began to emerge and this is known by the name of its natural gait—Paso Fino, or fine gait. These are the horses Columbus and the conquistadores brought to the new world. Paso Finos like Barbs have the characteristics of "primitive" horses: small round croup, low tail set, short thick neck, and the sub-convex facial profile. The nose turns down from the eyes to the nostrils like a ram's head.

This describes Genji perfectly. Over the years Genji's dapples and dorsal stripe have dissolved into white. His legs have some flecks of black, and his mane and tail are a mixture of black and white which looks gray.

When I do go to his stable, I groom him, saddle up and ride out the gate to the equestrian trail. I choose either going up toward Ojai, or down toward the ocean. He does very well on this trail considering that through a rail fence parallel to the equestrian trail is a paved bicycle path busy with bicycle riders, joggers, and dogs on leashes. Genji had spent six years riding out the ranch gate and into the surrounding Santa Fe National Forest with Rasa and Tara bounding along with us, so this is all new to him.

As seems to happen with animals, Genji reaches a tipping point physically and mentally that suddenly becomes evident. Tano, my farrier, who grew up in Columbia with Paso Finos, shows me the thrush in all four of Genji's hooves. He explains that it is even in the nail holes. Simultaneously, Genji has lost weight and I can tell that his hay is the issue, because the stable feeds low quality hay.

After the shoeing I go riding, or I think I will go riding. Genji won't move forward. He won't go past parked cars, under the bridge to the trail gate, across the creek a different direction for a shorter ride. Then he finally just stops and will not move one inch. I sit on him perplexed, feeling completely incompetent, and very concerned. In eleven years of riding him, he has never, ever not gone forward. If anything, my challenge is to slow him down as he gaits his way anywhere. I dismount and lead him back to the barn. I unsaddle him, groom him, and realize there is a major problem that needs to be identified and resolved.

I treat his hooves with an organic thrush product several times a week. I have his vet file his teeth, give him all of his vaccinations, and assess his physical condition. His weight loss is a concern with vertebrae beginning to protrude. I buy my own hay—orchard grass, what he has eaten until he moved to California from the high country. In the process of going to the barn to treat his hooves, I am there at different times of the day, and different days than when I had my specific schedule for riding. As a result I observe many things that I have never noticed at the stable. I see how the water container is dumped into the corral and has no way to drain out, so that Genji is always standing in mud. This explains the thrush. I tell Roberto, the employee there, the problem and have him dig a small ditch for the water to escape. I see how fast Pablo drives the cart into the barn and past Genji's stall. It is an electric cart and is recharged via a plug in the tack room directly across the aisle from his stall. This charging process makes an annoying sound. I see how the tools are leaned against the fence of Genji's corral, and how Roberto walks swiftly past the front of the barn and grabs a tool. This startles Genji. In fact everything I see going on around him makes him nervous. The employees wave their arms, move suddenly, talk loudly, and basically act like predators to the sensitive, highly developed flight instinct of a Paso Fino. And always droning in the background is the traffic on Highway 33 from Ventura to Ojai—semi-trucks, motorcycles, cars. Genji has really not been exposed to this level of sound in all of his life.

I give the stable my thirty day notice and I call Laura. I introduce Genji and Laura then we go outside the barn on the grass to talk. There are pepper trees, picnic tables, and the area is fenced.

"There was a snake in my corral and it scared me. They couldn't figure out what was wrong, so they took me out of my stall and bumped into me with the cart."

"I think Genji probably bumped into the cart because it takes up half of the aisle, and I'm sure that he was nervous and excited to have a stranger handle him."

"The truck parked there makes a big noise and scares me."

"He is referring to the manure truck, and Roberto had indeed told me the week before the shoeing about the incident with the truck not starting and in the attempt to start it, turning the key repeatedly, and Genji reacting to that. Tano had been told this same story by Roberto and had repeated it to me when he was shoeing Genji."

"The people here are empty."

"What do you mean by empty?" Laura asks.

"The people don't talk to us. I want to run and buck and roll."

We take Genji into the arena and turn him loose. We stand inside the arena near the gate. Genji gallops, kicks, bucks, and shakes his head. He runs up to us. I stroke his head then he runs off again. He finds a special place then rolls and rolls and rolls. He has one more gallop and returns to us. I put his halter on and we go back to his stall.

"Tell Genji that I love him and that I love riding him."

"I love you too. How are the dogs?"

"They've been sick, but they are better now."

"Oh, I was worried about them. I'm glad I haven't been sick."

As I put the halter and lead rope in the tack room, Genji says, "I miss you already."

I despair at how much I have neglected him while he has been quietly suffering at this stable. I thank Laura. We hug and leave.

I look at every stable in the valley. Nothing appeals. My three criteria are that there has to be access to trail riding without using a trailer, I want him to have a stall with a corral, and it has to be a non-dilapidated well run facility in a quiet location. I call Tano.

"I have looked at every stable and I don't like anything."

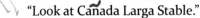 "Look at Cañada Larga Stable."

By now I have one week left of my thirty days. I call, get directions, and I drive out on a Sunday in the late afternoon. I've never driven on this road which is half-way between my home and the ocean. I am absolutely amazed. At the beginning of the road are several rustic homes close together, then an area with many horses in an assortment of corrals and funky stalls made of a variety of scrap wood. A row of pick-ups and SUV's are parked along the side of the road. Hispanic vaqueros are riding or standing around talking. I wave at them and recognize the horses from the Fourth of July parade. They ride Andalusians crossed with Quarter Horses that they call Aztecas, and train them to gait.

From there the valley spreads out in front of me—rolling hills covered with grass and chaparral, live oaks marching up the steep, narrow ravines. Black Angus graze on open ranchland. There are no houses, no buildings. I drive over a cattle guard where I see two cowboys riding their horses out in the pasture of cattle. I feel like I've entered a time warp. The road continues to wind to a gate. Forbidding large "No Trespassing" signs are posted. I get out of my car, open the gate, drive through, get out of my car and close the gate. I drive past a herd of free range horses and through the entrance of Canada Larga Stable. I know immediately that I have found Genji's new home.

Natasha, the manager, tells me to look around. She is a hot, sexy lady with a lion's mane of brown hair. She is dressed in minute shorts and a provocative low cut top, which reveals ample cleavage. My image of a stable manager is

Minutes FROM Beach + Downtown Ventura

instantly annihilated. I am in horse-owner heaven. There is a large covered riding arena, a dressage arena, a small covered riding arena, round pens, turn-out pens, a jumping arena in a former polo field, and four barns, plus a variety of separate corrals and paddocks. I eliminate the barn with the aisle because I think the aisle in Genji's present barn creates a lot of his nervousness. There is a small shed row barn that faces a lawn and the parking area. It has corrals on the back side which face the corrals from the large barn behind it, and it has a stall available. I choose that stall, but Natasha agrees to trade places with an empty stall on the end to one in the middle, because I also think that being on the end has caused problems for Genji. This little barn has six stalls, is framed on one end with a walnut tree and the other end with a pepper tree, plus has its own tack room. I tell Natasha I will have Genji there in three days.

I research supplements for hooves and nervousness, find a grain that is nutritious for a senior horse, and order three feedings a day of grass hay. I treat his hooves for the thrush and I don't ride him. I hand walk him everywhere. I need the exercise and he needs to explore his new surroundings with no pressure. I do this for a month. I turn him out in a large circular turn-out pen where he gallops, bucks, kicks, rolls and runs up to me with a snort and a loud nostril-flaring exhale. I try to imitate him and start to laugh. I cannot do that. I enjoy the participation in his turn-out. We play together.

Finally one day I decide that his feet are healing, he is gaining weight, he seems more relaxed, and I think it is time to go riding. I want a non-failure experience, so I walk him to the large riding arena to ride him there. He seems fine until I try to ride past the gate that opens between the arena and the aisle in Natasha's barn where her horses and horses she trains are kept. He stops and will not move. There are other riders in the arena and of course, I think I look like a fool, but I dismount and lead Genji back out.

For my second ride, I ride in the small covered arena. He does very well, but it is really too small for a gaited horse. We have our success, and I am determined to build on it. The next time I ride in the large arena, I avoid that gate. We ride the length of the center of the arena, and diagonally from corner to corner. He is fine with that. Next, I am there on a weekend when it is much busier at the stable. As I am saddling up, I see someone head for the gate and out on a trail. I decide to follow that horse and rider to give Genji some confidence about his new surroundings. It doesn't take long for us to catch up,

I introduce myself, explain the problem, and hooray! Genji is on a trail ride again. It is a challenge to ride a gaited horse with a non-gaited horse. They move much faster even at a basic walk. The *corto* gait is speedier and smoother than a jog or trot, and the *largo* gait is fast without having to gallop. So, you always have to turn around to talk, or stop and wait for the other horse and rider to catch up.

This ride got Genji out the gate and on the trail, but for me riding is not a social event. I like to ride alone so that the entire experience is between me and my horse. I like to observe the nature and landscape around me and enjoy the quiet of it except for the sound of Genji's hooves dancing along the ground. Genji is the kind of sensitive horse that if the rider's mind wanders and is no longer focused with him—he knows it, and that is when he jumps sideways, which immediately brings my attention back. My rides on Genji are deep meditations that clear my mind of the clutter that accumulates from everyday life.

So, when we can successfully go out the gate to ride by ourselves I know he is recovering from all of the stress, scariness, and feed issues that he experienced. I don't know if Genji knows the sound of my car, but he does know the sound of my footsteps, and as I walk from the car across the grass to his stall, he comes up to the stall door to greet me. I always call, "Geeeennjiii," making his name sound like a whinny. He always whinnies back.

I don't think that Genji can call the other horse owners here "empty people." The women with horses in his barn always ask me how he is doing and admit to giving him treats when they haven't seen me at the stable every day. So, I know there is a lot of horse love here. The stalls and corrals are meticulously clean, and the horses are fed three times a day, which is healthier for penned up grazing animals. I finally feel like I don't have to worry about his care anymore. When I leave after riding him I give him a few carrots and apples. "I love you." He extends his nose to me for a touch and goes back to the carrots and apples.

My heart always feels content and full when I drive back down the valley, sun lower in the sky, grasses becoming greener after an autumn rain.

11

Early one morning as I am looking up the hill behind the house, I see a small grayish animal hopping and bounding across the open space. I think it is a rabbit. Then a coyote comes out of the brush and starts trotting after it. I think, oh, the coyote is going to kill that rabbit. They both disappear into the bushes on the other side of the open space. I wait quietly. After a while they both appear going back across the hill together. A baby coyote! The smallest one I've ever seen. How special! The little guy is playing like a kitten on what might have been its first excursion out of the den. And, only one. There are usually two, so one must not have survived. I always keep an eye out for the little coyote, but it is a few months later before it re-appears.

Kundun and I are on the edge of the oak grove. He stands absolutely still, his big radar ears pointed toward the fence on the far side of the grove. He is alert. I follow his gaze with mine. Then I see a movement on the other side of the fence. Kundun, completely ignoring any arthritic pain, sprints across the space in a flash. He disappears into the bushes on this side of the wire fence. Then the coyote and Kundun play with each other by running back and forth with the fence between them. The coyote yips as they play. Soon the coyote disappears and Kundun returns with a big smile from ear to ear.

So, of course, when Laura comes, my first question is, "Kundun, how do you know you can trust that coyote?"

"I knew I could trust him when I saw his eyes. Now we are friends. The coyote would like water put out for him. Crush is very bored and needs an outing. It's really important to go to the grassy park and the ocean."

I had taken Rasa to a park in Ventura next to the ocean. Dogs aren't allowed on the state beach there, but the huge grassy area with trees and picnic sites between the 101 and the sand dunes does allow dogs. Rasa has obviously told Kundun about this place and her walk there.

"You should go to school to learn how to heal with your hands," Kundun adds.

"We can go to the beach now that my cancer is gone."

I've attempted a variety of walks with Rasa, and I usually always include Tara on walks with Rasa. Our walks are confined to weekdays because everybody—thirty million Californians—are out on weekends on the trails, at the parks, at the beach. Rasa is other dog aggressive and hates sharing as far as she can see with another dog. So, it's impossible to take her to most places. We have Santa Claus Beach in Carpenteria unless it is summer. We have the big grassy park by the beach in Ventura. We have the grounds at the Krotona Theosophical Society in Ojai. Hills are out, she can no longer manage them. Off leash is absolutely out of the question. She would leave a trail of mangled Chihuahuas and miniature poodles, but I'm sure she would try to take on large dogs as well—bears, coyotes, dogs—it's all the same to her. She's a tough girl and Tara is her back up.

On one of those attempted walks, the three of us were on the bicycle and equestrian trail that is the former railroad track from Ventura to Ojai. We were near Libby Park in Ojai. Suddenly Rasa rushed a pit bull behind a fence and pulled the leash out of my hands. As I tried to grab her leash while she and the pit bull were fighting through the fence, a second dog came up behind the fence and Tara took on that one. I could not pull Rasa and Tara away until finally the owner called her dogs. The physical effort of trying to collect my dogs gave me an asthma attack. So, we went back to the car and went home.

But Rasa is right. We need to take some walks. Finding a place to take walks is the challenge.

"I don't want Laura to get sad, and I will hug her when she is," Rasa says.

Laura explains, "When I was driving here, I was feeling sad because I just lost a kitty friend that belonged to a client."

Laura has told me in the beginning that if I got upset in the car like I did about Tara, the dogs would know because we are so connected.

"The day the workmen leave, Mom has got to start writing her book about healing dogs!" Kundun pronounces.

We have a construction project at our house that is driving us all crazy with the noise. During an intense winter rain, water cascaded in a waterfall through the tops of double French doors on the south side of the house and ruined the maple floor in that room. I had a temporary fix of plastic sheeting nailed over the doors, the doors nailed shut, and waited until May to begin the project. Because the weather comes from the south and the ocean, I decided to replace four sets of French doors on that side with windows and cover the porch with a roof. Also the floor in the flooded room had to be replaced, and while they were doing that, I had the floor raised six inches to eliminate a step on two sides of the room. Many days I put the dogs in the car to get them away from the noise and take them with me to do errands. The banging begins every morning at seven and doesn't stop until five. A three week job has turned into two months, and we are all fairly insane from it.

I ask Tara, "What is happening when your back legs shake and tremble?"

"They do this mostly at night," I explain to Laura.

"I get scared. It doesn't seem like my legs are connected to me when they shake sometimes. I realize I don't see as well as everyone else and I wonder if I will be normal. Knowing this makes me uncomfortable. I have to rely on other senses, as well as on my heart."

Rasa has two questions for me. "Do you walk with more awareness since I got sick? Do you believe that angels can enter the top of your head and give you ideas? I do!"

I have no answer for her right now, "I need to think about this."

12

Tara joins us now for our sessions with Cynthia. Her body works on adrenaline overload and her nervous system. She is happy to be included, and like Rasa and Kundun, lies down while the tuning fork is playing its mesmerizing melody. Eventually Tara begins to go behind Cynthia's desk to watch her and get petted. Both Rasa and Tara like to watch her while she very mystically moves her hands to test them. Since dogs are so much more aware of aspects beyond the skin boundary, I wonder what they perceive. They all definitely love her, and never let her forget the little delicious treat at the end of our sessions before we traipse down the stairs and out the door.

After my disappointment with the second kennel, I try Dog Friendly, which Laura recommends for Kundun. I call Kay to inquire about boarding.

"He has to come in for an interview first, so we need to make an appointment. I do interviews Friday, Saturday and Sunday mornings."

I make an appointment for the following Saturday morning and get directions. Kay's kennel is at her home, and it is the kind of kennel where all of the dogs are together. She has both daycare and overnight boarding. At night the boarders all go into her home where they sleep in cubicles. The two kennels that I have tried so far keep the dogs outdoors at night, and I don't like that. My dogs are used to being inside at night. The winters here are damp and chilly, so my quest has been for what in New Mexico is a typical kennel, and what in southern California seems to be an unusual kennel.

I get lost trying to find Kay's home. The directions are too vague for my literal mind. I finally call and by the time I arrive I am very late. The gate at the street is unlocked by Kay, a very dynamic woman with reddish hair who sizes up Kundun as he walks in. Kundun is shaking because he always shakes on the way into the vet, the groomer, and the kennel. Kay ushers us into a separate area from the dogs that are all together. We sit in an arrangement of patio furniture behind her home and talk.

"You can take his leash off."

Kundun begins to wander a little and sniff everything. He basically ignores all of the other dogs. As he sits next to Kay, he tucks his ears back against his head.

"See how he does this with his ears? He is part greyhound."

"I know he is part hound, but never would have guessed greyhound. He can run short distances very fast in spite of his bulky pit bull body. That's a great observation."

"I am a behaviorist."

We talk and she observes Kundun, as well as me I'm certain.

"I'd like him to come for day care for one day, so call me to make reservations." Kay walks us to the gate, unlocks it, and lets us out.

"Yay Kundun, you passed the interview!" I am totally relieved because by now I've run out of options for boarding. Kay will feed him his raw food diet and give him his medications. I'm beginning to realize that boarding options for senior dogs are limited. They have special diets, many supplements, and medications.

Dr. Alice cuts back Rasa's Leukeran—the oral chemo, and the prednisone, as well as the pepsid for stomach upset from the chemo. As she gets less and less prednisone, I begin to notice a funny gait emerge. When going downhill her front legs look like they are moving at twice the speed of her back legs, and taking smaller steps. She moves stiffly and no longer jumps off the wall that skirts the courtyard plus flanks the hillside separating the wild from the tended gardens surrounding the house.

Dr. Jill at Buena recommends that Kundun get acupuncture for his arthritis. She sends us to Dr. Karen Martin in Thousand Oaks. I make an appointment for both Rasa and Kundun. She is booked weeks in advance. It's approximately a thirty to forty minute drive from my home to her clinic.

The East/West Clinic waiting room is busy. There are old dogs that can barely walk. There is a dog that looks like it has hip dysplasia. There are small dogs being carried. Every dog has a mobility issue. Kundun appears to have minor problems compared to other patients. We are ushered into a spacious room with a curved wall of glass bricks. Eventually Dr. Karen opens the door, peeks in, then goes up to Kundun and kneels on the floor next to him. She pets and rubs him, and feeds him some treats. Attractive and young looking, Dr. Karen is almost elfish as she lovingly interacts with Kundun. He immediately loves her.

I tell her Rasa's story, and as she rubs and pets Rasa, she explains, "Mast cells love electricity, and acupuncture needles create electricity, so Rasa should never have acupuncture." She runs her hand down Rasa's back and determines that it is her shoulders that have an issue. This explains her odd gait that the prednisone was masking.

"Let's just say that she was a hard hitting dog."

She begins to unwrap sterilized needles, and taps them in—a few on Kundun's head, pairs of them along his back, and a couple in his back legs. She has a soft rug for the dogs to lie on, and there is a continuous supply of treats coming out of her pocket. After Kundun looks like a porcupine she leaves the room. Kundun is surprisingly good about lying quietly for twenty or thirty minutes with needles sticking out everywhere.

On the drive back home the words "hard hitting" keep echoing in my mind. I visualize Rasa running at top speed along the fence, which paralleled the driveway at the ranch, then jumping up against the perpendicular end of the fence hitting it hard with her front feet, back legs springing up and hitting the fence as well, and doing this repeatedly as well as barking like crazy when anyone would drive up the road. Little did I realize what the long term effects of this would be from doing it for eight years. She also jumped down from rocks and cliffs on hikes. Rasa has always been an athletic girl.

After meeting Dr. Karen, I begin to give Rasa acupressure massage from her ears to her tail every night. She loves it and hopefully it is relieving some of her pain. I can't leave Tara out, so she gets an acupressure massage as well. Kundun begins a regular regimen of acupuncture. He appears to love it. He gets very excited as soon as we turn into the parking lot. It does seem to help, and I maintain the schedule for several months.

The young little coyote appears regularly on the hill above the house. Sometimes he even trots on top of the low rock wall behind the black chain link fence on the uphill side of the dog yard. I've seen him peek his head around the end of the wall and look down into the kitchen. Of course, as soon as the dogs know he is there, they dash out the door barking. Kundun doesn't bark at him, because they are friends. The coyote backs off twenty feet or so, sits down and yips right back at the dogs.

At night after we are in bed, I can hear the coyote making his way to San Antonio Creek. Every yard he passes that has dogs becomes a barking chorus.

But the coyote doesn't keep going. He stops at every place and yips right back at the dogs. I think it is very funny, so I start calling him Chatty, because he chats it up with all of the canines in the neighborhood. He has a very distinctive yip and I recognize it even in his pack when they hunt.

One day I am out with Kundun. I stand near the garage while he is standing alert on the edge of the slope going down into the oak grove. All of a sudden he dashes into the trees. Coming the other direction running is Chatty. They have a game of circling the giant oaks. Then Chatty cuts diagonally out of the trees and into the front yard with Kundun right behind him. I move from the garage to the top of the driveway so I can see them. There is a large pile of river rocks in the center of the yard. First they run one direction Chatty in front and Kundun chasing around the pile. Then they turn and run the other direction Kundun in front and Chatty chasing. Around and around they run. I have never seen a wild animal and a domestic one play together. I had no idea Kundun could even run like that anymore. Apparently they say goodbye and Chatty runs one direction while Kundun comes up the driveway with a big grin on his face.

He can barely move for the next week.

13

It is early October and I take Rasa and Tara on a road trip north to visit my sister in Napa. Kundun goes to stay with Kay. On this drive I decide to drive on 101, or as it is called in California, the 101. The 101 winds along the coast from Ventura to Santa Barbara. Sometimes the Channel Islands to the west are crystal clear, usually the day following a rain, but most of the time they are hidden in the ocean mist and fog. From Santa Barbara the 101 winds along the coast but is high above cliffs before it climbs over the coastal range into rolling hills covered with live oaks on the way to San Luis Obispo. The grassy hills are already turning green with early rains this year. Cows graze and there are a few small groups of deer.

The 101 follows El Camino Real, the original path of the Spanish conquistadores and priests. It passes through Paso Robles, past the old San Miguel Mission, and north along the Salinas River to Salinas. There it transforms from a four-lane to an eight-lane to accommodate commuters going to and from Silicon Valley. The valley is wide here with miles of agricultural activity, which disappears into the populated and busy bay area south of San Jose.

When we arrive at the ranch, Rasa and Tara are very excited to be there, so I put them in the fenced yard. Within seconds Rasa has raced across the lawn, grabbed and killed a ground squirrel and is eating it. This will definitely put her in good favor with my brother-in-law, who isn't real crazy about my dogs, but who hates the ground squirrels, and takes shots at them regularly with a rifle.

Unfortunately before I left home Genji stepped on my right foot. It was completely my fault. I was leading him and turned my upper body to say something to someone. Genji followed my turn, however with my feet still facing forward his hoof came down on me. I have a huge bruise, and can barely walk. The only shoes I can wear are Teva sandals with socks. This eliminates being able to hike on any trails, so Rasa, Tara and I walk on flat dirt and paved roads that wind around the property. They continuously lunge and pull trying to smell all of the scents along the way, and of course, wanting to run and track whatever it is—I can't let them do that. They don't know they are eleven years old. The terrain is steep, rocky and covered with dense chaparral. If anything would happen to one of them I simply would never find her. With the wild pigs, coyotes, bobcats, and a mountain lion here, I keep them leashed and penned.

We return home after about twelve days. I have enjoyed wineries and excellent restaurants. Rasa and Tara have enjoyed a big lawn and much running and barking at all of the ranch activities.

The morning after arriving home, I see a dead rat in a stone planter in the outdoor entry from the driveway in front of the garage inside a wrought iron gate. It's possible that it could have climbed in, although at first I think it is a bad joke perpetrated by Daniel. I put on my rubber gloves, put it in the garbage, and think it is odd, but that is all. I observe that it appears to be recently dead. The next day Cassidy comes to visit, and as we are walking out the back door and toward the entry gate that evening, there is a small mouse shaking and wobbling in the throes of death. I get it now—they've been poisoned! I scoop up the mouse and tie it up in a small plastic bag. This suffocates them fairly quickly, and I toss it in the garbage. I look all around this courtyard, the front of the garage and the upper driveway area. I find nothing. We go to dinner and when we return it is dark.

In the morning I am in the courtyard off the kitchen where the dogs are when they are outside. As I am watering, I see a dead rat by one of the dog beds. It absolutely was not there two days before, but I didn't notice anything yesterday. The rat is not freshly dead, is decomposing, and looks like it could have teeth marks, but it's hard to tell. I am furious at myself for not seeing this sooner. I get rid of it and walk over every inch of the dog yard looking for dead rodents—nothing.

I have no idea whether Rasa or Tara got to this rat, but I begin to keep a close watch on both of them. One night later Tara jumps off the bed in the middle of the night. We have a drill for this I grope for the light switch on the lamp cord next to my bed, turn the nightstand light on, grab my bathrobe, and we run out of the bedroom, down the hall as I frantically turn on light switches guided by night lights in every outlet along the way. We fly down the stairs, careen through the kitchen, then I unlock and open the door to the courtyard, plus flip on the outside lights for the dog, that like me cannot see well in the dark. Next I go through the living room and into an adjoining room to turn on more outside lights so that Tara can see where she is going.

Kundun knows all is not well and nervously watches from his bed in the kitchen. Tara comes back to the kitchen door. I have put a large potty pad on the floor as the rule is that when you jump off the bed in the middle of the night—you stay in the kitchen for the rest of the night. She curls up in her bed. I pet her, leave the light over the stove on low, and return to the bedroom turning off the lights on the way back. I can't sleep. I need to go out in the yard and see what happened when it is light. I am terrified for my precious Tara.

In the morning as soon as it is barely light I rush to the kitchen. Tara is still alive, but I know she has been poisoned by the rat poison in the dead rat I found two days before. A trip outside in the dawn dressed in my bathrobe and slippers to the area where I saw her in the night reveals a bright red bloody, mucous-like pool of diarrhea. After feeding the dogs in the morning, Tara runs out the door and I follow to see a pile of bloody vomit. This is bad and it is Sunday. The vet is closed. I am reluctant to take her to the emergency vet in Oxnard. Tara is used to the people at Buena, and I trust them with her sensitive emotions and fear. I make a risky decision. We go through the same routine Sunday night, and Monday morning at eight I call Buena to make an emergency appointment. I arrive with Tara an hour later.

She is given a vitamin K shot to clot the blood because rat poison causes internal bleeding, which is what kills rodents that ingest it, and consequently anything that ingests them. She is given metronidazole for diarrhea, and sucralfate which is dissolved in water to coat the stomach and intestinal linings.

Now my personal paranoia about people trying to harm my dogs gushes to the surface. I left a man in charge of watering plants in the courtyards for me while Rasa, Tara and I were gone. He has done handyman type work for me since I moved in two years ago. In the past four months Daniel has become strange and incompetent. I'm now convinced he poisoned the rats. My daughter tells me, "Mom he's weird, but he's not a sociopath." With my past experience with employees and my horse and dogs, I'm not convinced. I fire Daniel, change my gate code, lock myself in my house and focus on taking care of Tara. The dogs are not allowed to go outside without me, and I continuously patrol for dead rodents. No more appear.

I reflect on the utterly bizarre past ten year history of living alone, having protective dogs and the endless repeated situations of employees and hired workers brutalizing my dogs. I think there is a hidden societal agenda about women who live alone, and something not being "normal" about that. When I was young these women were referred to as spinsters and old maids. Then society changed—women got divorced, worked, and lived alone. Women changed—they worked out, became athletic, pursued educations and careers.

In New Mexico many of the Spanish who settled there in the seventeenth century escaped the Spanish Inquisition. This included Jews who were forced to convert to Christianity or be tortured and killed. They are Sephartic Jews from the regions of Spain and Portugal. Their descendants are Christians, but they follow many Jewish traditions that lost their religious meaning over the centuries. Manys of these people fled Spain, sailed to Mexico and made the journey up the Rio Grande Valley into what is now northern New Mexico. I have a completely unfounded theory that like the now meaningless rituals moved forward in time for over four hundred years, ugly belief remnants also exist in the post-Inquisition memory. We know that women who lived alone on the physical edge of European communities, and who had knowledge of herbs and healing, as well as had cats for pets were persecuted by the Christian Church as witches.

I was always asked the same question by Norteno men, "Aren't you afraid to live out here alone?"

My two hundred acres was an in-holding, completely surrounded by the Santa Fe National Forest. I had a few neighbors, but we lived with the same philosophy—I moved out here for privacy.

My response to this question was always, "No."

One day I picked up a young man who was walking on the dirt road I lived on, and who lived beyond my gate. We passed a certain place and I said, "I saw a black bear right there a few days ago."

"What did it do run away?"

"No, actually we looked at each other for a while, and then it ambled up the hill."

Jaime simultaneously threw his back against the passenger door, grabbed the handle of the door, and moved as far away from me as possible in the confined area of the truck cab. With big brown eyes he asked, "What are you a *bruja*?"

I finally understood the issue. A *bruja*, a witch—I'm a witch. You can't burn them at the stake now, but you can terrorize their dogs. I rather liked being considered a *bruja*. It elevated me on the power scale. I didn't need to worry about not having a gun—I could just cast spells.

When Rasa and Tara were one year old I moved to my ranch full time. The work was still ongoing at the house on the exterior. The logs were sandblasted, decks rebuilt, chinking redone. Several times I left them in their pen with Kabuki while I went into Santa Fe to do errands and undergo extensive dental work. Workmen were there when I left and gone when I returned. Kabuki would be mysteriously outside of the pen. The dogs were always excited to see me, and I did not realize what a cruel, perverted torture routine was occurring while I was gone. They are my dogs, puppies still in their own pen at their own home. I believed people were intrinsically good, that I could leave my dogs safely at home alone without my being there.

Rasa and Tara weren't completely trained to use the outdoors when they needed to pee or poop. Their expansive yard that I had fenced for them was ready, however workmen needed access to do exterior work on my house. I had the doors and windows closed in the house because of the dust created by the work. The house was airless and hot and I thought leaving them inside in crates would be dangerous. Little did I realize.

I didn't know that the workmen were sadistically abusing my dogs. It was beyond my comprehension that someone would do this to eleven or twelve month old puppies at their own home. Rasa and Tara began to exhibit serious behavior problems. They became unexplainably aggressive. I enrolled Tara in a fear-based aggression class still not understanding what had happened.

Then one day during the following winter approximately five months later I had two friends visiting. One of them picked up a fleece ball to throw to Tara to play with her. I saw the look of absolute terror on Tara's face as my friend's arm went up, but before I could say stop, the ball hit her on her back as she dived into her crate. In that instant I realized what had happened. I flashed back on the rocks in the dog yard that were mysteriously roundish and hand-size that I would find when I cleaned up the poop. I didn't get it then but now I did.

Now I understood everything.

Tara was melt-down terrified of hoses, ropes, rakes, shovels, the sound made by a ladder or an ironing board opening or closing, and any kind of vacuum, lawnmower, or weed-whacker sound sent her into hiding. She was so completely emotionally and psychologically devastated by her experience I wasn't sure she could survive to act even semi-normal. In fact I wondered if she would ultimately have to be euthanized. The contractor accused me of lying, said his men loved dogs. There was no animal abuse law in place in New Mexico at the time or I would have filed charges. But there was an eye witness who came forward months later, so eventually I knew it had happened.

Rasa became extremely aggressive. She would try to go through car windows if a man came anywhere near the car. She growled and snarled at everything and everyone, sometimes even me. Tara received the main focus of this mindless, hateful, mean violence because I think Rasa went into the one dog house, and Tara was left at the mercy of vicious, savage men. My belief that people are intrinsically good, that I could trust workmen with my dogs at home that this kind of behavior did not exist in my realm, my innocence—all of it was shattered. The very standard for my interacting with other humans, the loving kindness I had been taught by my grandmother was destroyed. As I embraced my land, nature, and my solitary lifestyle, I became more and more suspicious and paranoid of people, and more protective of my dogs.

I dearly loved Tara and I was determined to rehabilitate her as best as I could. I threw out all of the dog training rules—they don't work with abused dogs. I now had a fearful aggressive dog—Tara, and an irrational aggressive dog—Rasa. I began to try to rehabilitate them without even knowing what I was doing. I used lots of love and patience with all positive reinforcement. I could not wipe their eyes or even touch their heads. They growled at me. Everything had to be positive from my end or I would get nowhere. Every day I took a Kleenex and quickly touched their noses. They growled. I said, "Good girl!" Somehow we worked our way to wiping eyes, lifting up and looking in ears, feeling legs and paws, being petted, hugged and loved. Whatever little progress there was even if it included growling, they got a "Good girl!" I was enthusiastic no matter how disappointed I felt and I celebrated quietly for any improvement whatsoever. I enrolled Tara in a trick class. She loved it and learned tricks easily. I taught Rasa and by then Kundun tricks also, but Tara was the only one that learned roll-over and roll-over again, as well as shake—then other paw.

It was one year before I could reach out and touch my own dog. That is how terrified Tara was. I was angry. I was sad. I was dumbfounded at my own inability to see what was happening. I began to take Tara with me on road trips from Pecos to Durango, Colorado where I went for business and on one trip to Moab, Utah where my family had a reunion. We had our own little log cabin there which she guarded during the day from her vantage point on the sofa, and she cuddled with me on the bed at night. I think these special journeys did more for her than anything else. We were in the pick-up cab for hours together, took walks, slept together and it all made her feel loved and safe. We developed a bond that became deep and a special love grew between us.

She began to greet me again with her dolly in her mouth, which evoked me to give her what I called a dolly girl hug. I sat on a step usually and she would walk around my back. As she came up to my side I would put my arm around her and give her a hug. She repeated this over and over. Slowly Tara began to emerge from the darkness of her mental hell. She remained timid, shy, and frightened of men. But the precious cuteness and playful attitude found its way back into our lives. After four years Tara was doing very well.

When I hired Jake and Karen to be caretakers and live in the apartment over the garage I entrusted the care of my animal family to these people— two cats, three dogs, and two horses. After the incident with Tara while I was traveling in Burma I decided to fire Jake and Karen, but it was almost Christmas and I have a heart, a conscience, and I'm a nice person. So, in February I gave them a five month notice to be fair, and very frankly that was my mistake. Again, I could not fathom these people abusing my dog. Oh, they liked Kundun and Rasa—they were normal dogs. But Tara was different and they picked on her. So, while I was gone on two business trips and to a family reunion Tara was abused by Karen. By the end of it all Tara was hiding under the deck terrified, shaking, and unable to even come to me. She was afraid to come in the door of the house. She would look up at my arm holding the door open then run. Obviously she had had the door slammed in her face repeatedly, probably wasn't allowed in the house to eat or for the night. She also developed a fear of rugs being shaken. There was a rug just outside the door which was one of her favorite places to lie. I couldn't touch a rug anymore without her running away. There was no aspect of her life that had not become a fearful experience. Square one had become the sole square. I started over with the shattered pieces of her mind.

It was two and one-half years after Jake and Karen left when I moved to California. Only in a new house with a different door did Tara let go of her fears. And in California I became monster mom to my dogs. What I lost was any innocent belief in people generally being intrinsically good. Any one on my property was a potential dog abuser. I literally went outside with each dog one at a time for potty breaks when workmen were around. And was I being too paranoid? No! While I was outside with Rasa a worker jumped over the fence right in front of me with a large cardboard tube in his hands. I knew what that tube was for—hitting a dog. I got Rasa in the house, marched out and found who the worker was—on the roofing crew, called the owner of the roofing business, and told him that I couldn't afford an altercation between one of my dogs and a workman. This was a polite way to make sure I never saw the guy again, which I didn't.

Basically Californians are nice people. They know a Catahoula when they see one, "Oh wow, are those Catahoulas?" But I never let anyone pet or touch them.

14

Within a week Tara has mostly recovered from the rat poison incident. Laura comes for a visit.

Rasa speaks up first, "I'm worried about Tara. I don't want anyone to die. I know about the bear."

I ask, "What bear?"

"You don't know about the bear? A bear wandered into Ojai and climbed up into a tree. The Fish and Game tranquilized it, which caused it to fall to the ground, and then they euthanized it," Laura explains.

"How do you know about this Rasa?"

"The coyotes told me."

Kundun speaks up, "I had to go to jail."

Laura and I look at each other and I start to laugh. "I pay forty dollars a day for him to stay at this ritzy kennel with Kay, and he thinks he is in jail?"

"They like me there, but I want to go on the trip."

I explain, "Kundun breathes all of the oxygen in the car, pants, drools, and is not a good traveler. He also poops on my sister's carpet. He can't go with us."

Kundun immediately changes the subject, "I want big chunky things in my food like dog treats. I'm sick of animals feeling like they're going to die. I want to see our horse. I didn't know people could die."

Laura and I had briefly spoken about Kay who had surgery for ovarian cancer. I'm taken by Kundun's idea that humans are immortal.

Now Rasa adds, "I want to see our horse also. If Tara dies, I'll die because I'll miss her too much. I need crystals in my head."

Laura gets a clarification about the crystals.

"I need crystals closer to my head than the bio-pad. I need some crystal energy."

"I have lots of crystals!" I pull out two and place one on each side of the inside of the large wicker looking crate where the bio-pad is always on, and the crate door is always open. Rasa goes into the crate and lies down with her head next to and in between the crystals.

"I can feel the crystal energy. Put one on top of the crate too."

I place two smaller crystals on top then she gets up and leaves the crate. Apparently she is happy with the results.

"A bear told me about the bear in Ojai being killed," Tara says.

"When does the bear talk to you?" Laura asks.

"A bear comes to talk to me at every half-moon. The bear talks to me because I can see its skull, and it knows I won't hurt it."

"How do you feel now?"

"I don't feel like I am going to die now. I licked something off a bush in the yard."

Laura and I decide that the cat mint and grass she eats tasted bad due to her illness.

Rasa advises me, "Mom needs to do stretching and breathing exercises. It will make her feel better. We love her so much now. We loved her before because we needed her, but now we love her for who she is."

I, of course, am overwhelmed by this expression of devotion. "Have any coyotes died from the poison?"

"Yes, one coyote died."

"Oh no, is it Kundun's friend Chatty?"

"No, he didn't die. They all know about the rats now."

"Play more music!" Rasa exclaims.

Our session ends, and I ponder the inter-species communication between domestic animals and wild animals. This is very mystical to me, and I become more curious about that aspect of our dialogue than who killed the rat to try to solve the source of the poisoning. Rasa said that she killed the rat, but she didn't get poisoned—Tara did. Sometimes our conversations aren't very empirical, much like talking to young children.

We live approximately five miles from where the bear was killed. It happened near the center of town where the Sunday Farmer's Market is held. So, I'm very interested in how this story moved from the site of the incident to my dog yard. And, Rasa and Tara were out of town when it happened. Kundun was across the Ventura River on the other side of the valley with Kay.

I don't know where the bear tree is located, but on Sunday I park my car and walk to the Farmer's Market. In a front yard I see a shrine at the base of a large pine tree. I stop. There are candles, flowers, and an assortment of cute stuffed teddy bears. There is an enlarged color photograph of the bear alive in this same tree. An artist who lives across the street has made a metal shield and placed it in the tree where the bear sat on a branch before being shot with the tranquilizer.

I feel terrible for the bear, because I love bears. The size and look of it in the photo remind me of the bear Rasa and Tara treed on the land in New Mexico at the beginning of a hike. I heard them barking crazily, and rushed up the side of the canyon above the creek to where they were jumping up on the trunk of a large ponderosa pine. I looked up and there was the bear standing with its back feet on one branch, and its upper body and front legs leaning over a higher branch looking down at the commotion. He was drooling in fear, and seemed young enough to me to possibly have a mother nearby. However, I took the time to look at the size of his feet, so that I would know the next time I saw tracks just what size of a bear made them. I immediately changed our hiking route, and called my hounds away from all of the excitement of treeing their first bear.

At the end of our hike back at the house, I saw a small gash on Tara's head. I guessed that she had been so close to the bear that one of its hind feet caught the top of her head on its way up the tree.

15

On November seventh I attend the bear dance at Casa de la Luna. People begin to gather at dusk bringing chairs or blankets. We sit around a large circle on the grass defined by tall slender willow branches in the ground. The branches are stripped of leaves and smaller branches except for the tops. The four directions are marked with their representative colors, red, yellow, black and white. In the center is a circular pile of dirt with two eagle feathers hanging on a short stake. People are quiet. In the lingering last light in the sky above three great egrets fly overhead. I wonder if anyone sees them except me. No one is looking up. I find this to be a very auspicious omen.

The eagle feathers are removed and the fire-builders begin to build the fire. Each person who enters through the doorway facing east is smudged with sage then makes a clockwise turn in the doorway when entering. Two men stand at this portal holding smoking sage during the entire ceremony. Each person also makes a small clockwise turn when leaving and is smudged then as well. Since I unknowingly placed my chair near the east portal, I was blessed with sage smudge for hours. The sage in California is different than in New Mexico. It's a bluish green color like the high country sage, but it has a wider leaf and smells different. Bundles of sage are continuously added to the fire, so that the smell of the cedar burning and the sage envelope the entire area. As I watch the fire burn, I think of all of my campfires in New Mexico—the ones outside my tipi when I slept there, and the ones in Hawk's Meadow when I had family for a barbeque, or just sat there by myself enjoying the dark, the quiet, and the stars. Of everything about my land, I think that I miss those campfires the most.

The first dancers are Aztec, Danza Azteca Mexicah de Ojai Bajo la Palabra de la Quinto Sol, with feather headdresses and costumes that glitter and sparkle in the firelight. Their dance is very animated. They are all women, so I wonder if their dance has something to do with the moon because they make me think of moonlight dancing in the night. After this dance four Chumash elders enter the circle and each stands facing the fire plus one of the directions. They make offerings to the spirit of the bear that was killed. They each throw tobacco, pour honey from a jar, and toss a plate of berries into the fire. For a moment I can smell the berries pungent in the air. The fire-builders place more wood on the fire. It is a large fire, but I cannot feel the warmth of it. I am bundled up, but am beginning to feel a chill. The nights have become cooler now, around fifty degrees.

The drummers enter the circle. I have noticed the chairs set up around a large cottonwood drum earlier. The drummers are all large Native men. I realize how the Pueblo Feast Days with their drumming and dancing became so much a part of my life in New Mexico, and I have missed it here. The Native culture is hidden in California. The fire-builders and the drummers are from the Barbareno-Ventureno Band of Mission Indians of the local Chumash tribe. The Chumash lived along the south central coast of California from Malibu to San Luis Obispo. They invented the plank canoe, were hunters and gatherers, and had a trade network from the Channel Islands to the higher altitude pine forests. Their way of life reflected the natural world around them. The word Ojai means moon, or moon's valley in the Chumash language. The Ojai Valley runs east and west, which is very unusual. It is still considered a sacred place to the Chumash people.

The drumbeat begins—not a heartbeat drumbeat—ta dum, ta dum like Pueblo drumbeats, but an earth shaking boom, boom, boom. A single dancer enters naked except for a loincloth and black feathers on his back and down his arms. Like a raven he prances, twirls, hops, and while he is doing this, explains to us, "I was born here in Ojai, the valley of the moon. This is a very powerful place. The bear spirit came to us in the sweat lodge. We are honoring Elliot/ Suawasuniset who gave his life on October tenth. The bear dance has not been danced for one hundred years in the Ojai Valley."

He dances out of the circle. Everything becomes very quiet and still. The fire is fed, crackles, and sends up a shower of bright sparks.

Mysteriously the bear dancers quietly gather to enter the circle. I turn to look. The crashing drumbeat begins. One by one the bears are smudged, turn one clockwise circle and begin to move around the fire. The raven dancer joins them. The full bear skins with heads seem eerily real. One of the bears makes bear noises. The dancers are stooped over and move purposefully. There is no pattern to the dance. They are bears wandering randomly. The bear dance appears to affect two of the bears physically. They are immediately tended to with sage smudge and eagle feathers. The bear dancers physically process the sickness and pain in the community from the shooting death of the bear. The sage cleanses them from the illness they are helping to transmute. The dance ends with members of the community invited to join in for a round dance.

The bear incident caused a community outpouring of anger toward the California Department of Fish and Game by local citizens who felt helpless to save the bear.

Laura was called to communicate with Elliot in the tree, "When I was told that Fish and Game had been called, I immediately began to prepare Elliot for death. I told him that his mother was waiting for him in Heaven. I told him to go up fast through all of the levels when he dies."

The Fish and Game decision was based on one operative. This happened during bear hunting season, bears are considered a food source, and a bear with highly potent sedatives in its system cannot be released into the wild. Apparently there is no effort to have alternative methods, such as used by the Bear League of Lake Tahoe. The Bear League supervises clearing the area of people, placing dogs inside, leaving a clear path for escape, and giving the bear time to feel safe and leave. The outrage in the Ojai Valley did channel into forming the Ojai Wildlife League (OWL) to deal with situations like this in the future.

16

After six months of going through layer after layer with Genji, I feel that I have finally pinpointed his physical problem. There was the weight loss from the low quality hay at his previous stable. I tried each one of the three kinds of hay the stable fed then decided to purchase my own grass hay. At the new stable I pay extra to have him fed grass hay three times a day. I feed him grain, and change the grain brand three times trying to get what works best. Genji gains weight with his new diet. The thrush clears up in three hooves, but not his left hind hoof.

The psychological damage is probably the worst issue. Genji became traumatized by the craziness at the last stable. This was multi-faceted in that there had been a terrible flood several years prior to Genji's arrival there, or even our move to California. The San Antonio Creek flooded and the entire stable which is located in the flood zone was under several feet of water. The story that I was told by several different people was that the stable did not notify horse-owners for three days. The rescue efforts were heroic and dangerous. I was told by a woman whose husband was attempting to rescue horses, of being in chest high water with logs swirling dangerously everywhere. Humans may think that an event like this doesn't affect horses. However the fear permeates everything. A horse told Genji, "When it rains kick your way out and run!" This fear was embedded in the stable and affected every horse whether a new arrival or one there during the flood.

Laura arrives for a conversation.

"I want to find out why Genji won't go up steep hills when we ride. He stops and won't move forward, I'm puzzled and concerned."

"They bumped into me with the cart. I have a pain that goes from my left hip along my back and down my right front leg ending behind my knee. It also goes up my neck on my right side. When I go downhill the pain is in my poll between my ears and my jaw."

"Wow, I can't even figure out how he goes riding. All of this and he does not favor a leg, is not lame, and his gait is completely smooth. What a horse! Obviously he rides for me and the love of riding. Very stoic, very brio. It makes me love him even more."

Genji is nibbling on some green grass near the small covered riding arena. A mare and her owner walk over to where we are. This horse was at the same previous stable for six days and was moved due to poor feed, behavior change, and abuse from employees. The mare tells Genji, "You are beautiful. I love your mane."

Genji replies, "I love your long legs, I wish sometimes that I had long legs."

"Oh Genji, you don't need long legs. You cover more ground faster than any horse I've known, and you are passionate about being ridden by me."

"Tell us a story," Laura says.

"There is a fox that gets on the barn roof."

Laura looks at me quizzically and I say, "Grey foxes climb trees. Red foxes were imported from England for fox hunts because indigenous American grey foxes when chased ran up into trees."

"How do you know about the fox on the roof?"

"The other horses told me."

"Genji, how do you like it here?" Laura asks.

"This place is like being in front of Heaven's Gate."

"Are you going to Heaven?"

"No. I think this place has helped Mom too. I want you to come out and read a book to me about horses. I want the dogs to come for a visit also."

This takes me back to Kundun's comment that, "I want to visit our horse too." I never ever thought of Genji as being "our." This is where human ego preconceptions meet other species' reality based concepts. Wow, our horse. I love it. Rasa and Tara went on every ride when we lived in New Mexico. Of course, he is our horse. Kundun walked to the barn with me every afternoon to feed the horses and he got a handful of grain treat in the process. Obviously Genji is not my horse—he is our horse! How could I not understand that?

Genji tells Laura repeatedly that he wants more moisture in his grain. I put his supplements in his grain and because they are in a powder form I can see how it seems dry and needs moisture. His grain and supplements are placed in a separate ziplock bag for each day of the week. Eventually I find out that every horse in his barn gets water in their supplements, I just needed to ask. Sometimes I simply cannot grasp protocol.

"Are you having stomach pain?" Genji asks me.

"I have been but it is better now."

"You should eat mashed herbs in butter."

Laura and I laugh a lot during these conversations. "Do you remember when Rasa and Kundun both wanted something from deep in the earth to make them feel better? I thought they meant something to eat. At some point after that Rasa had me arrange the crystals in the crate for her head. Crystals are from deep in the earth, so who knows? When Rasa asked me if I walk more carefully now since she got sick, I thought she meant the cancer and I was unable to connect the dots. One day I was walking in the field next door looking carefully at the ground and it struck me that Rasa meant after the spider bite."

A few months before Rasa's cancer tumor appeared, I had left her in the yard while I went to lunch with visiting family and friends on a Saturday. That evening I noticed a lump on her head above her left eye. It was curious but I had no idea what had caused it. In the morning on Sunday the lump had become larger and swollen which caused her eye to be partially closed. Of course these things always happen on weekends. I decided that she would have to go to Buena early Monday. By Monday morning her eye was completely closed and the lump had burst open and was oozing blood. She was shaking her head and blood was flying everywhere. I called Buena as soon as they opened, made an emergency appointment and ran up to my closet to grab a pair of panty hose. I cut off one leg and the foot of that leg then pulled it over her head to keep the blood contained. She did look funny. It was diagnosed as a brown recluse spider bite and necrosis had already begun. These are vicious spiders and their bites can cause the loss of limbs, or even death. I'd never heard of them before moving to California, but now I'd almost lost my dog to one of the critters. Rasa recovered with massive doses of anti-histamines, but it is my opinion that the flood of histamines in her blood from the bite probably is what activated the histamine loving mast cells that caused her cancer. Yes, I certainly do walk more carefully now. I shake out my boots and shoes before I wear them also.

It's as if the animals speak in *koans*, and one must meditate on the meaning, much like a zen master teaches students.

At the end of our session Laura asks, "What do you want to say for my blog?"

I say,"Genji is a happier horse because of Laura."

Then she asks Genji, "What do you want to say for my blog?"

"I am a happier horse because of my Mom."

17

"If I were a bear, I'd live inside the house not outside the house," Tara exclaims.

"I don't know why she said that," Rasa states.

"Have you talked to the bear, Tara?" I ask.

"The bear came and told me that it's time to hibernate, but it doesn't feel like it. I told the bear, well then don't do it! The bear asked if my mom knew if bears were large or small. I told the bear my mom knows bears are all sizes."

"When does the bear come talk to you?"

"She shows me a sunrise that looks like a sunset—do you have those here?"

"Actually we do have beautiful pink and red sunrises."

"Do you think this is a real bear?" Laura asks.

"No, I think it is a shaman bear. I've never seen bear scat here."

"My sister wants to have a baby. If she has a baby I'll get to look at it and it will smell neat. Tell Cassidy to say, 'Moon, get me pregnant.'" Rasa interjects.

"Tara will eat the baby," Kundun adds.

Laura looks horrified. I laugh, "Rasa licks her puppy dolly like a real puppy. She holds it down with her paw like I've seen dog moms do."

"They come alive when she isn't looking," Rasa says.

"Wasn't there a movie about this?"

"Genji says that he wants to live in the house. I told him, you can't live in the house—Mom would have to clean up your poop!" Kundun tells us.

"When did Genji tell you this?" Laura asks.

"After dinner we all mind-speak."

I look at Kundun. I look at Laura. "Wait a minute, these guys are all talking to each other telepathically?!"

Laura nods her head up and down—she knows all about this.

"Genji wants to know if I see Laura more than him. I said how would I know?"

"How is Chatty?" I ask Kundun. "What does he say?"

"Chatty is very sad. His mom died. She died in the den. They don't know what to do with her body. Chatty tried to pull her out, but couldn't. Four coyotes live in the den together."

"Where is their den?"

"He isn't allowed to say, but it is two driveway lengths away."

"How is your arthritis, Kundun?"

"Love dissolves all pain. I don't want to talk about being sick, because, it makes it worse."

"How do you know that?" Laura asks.

"I'm good at watching energies, and if someone drinks a hot drink and thinks it's making them better, it does."

"That's what I did last night. I drank hot tea because I wasn't feeling right and then I felt better."

"Dogs should sleep on people's beds and people should sleep on dog beds. Mom needs to do stretching exercises," Kundun adds.

"I'm getting a mat for stretching—it's on its way. Let's talk about the thunder, and how it scares Tara."

"Thunder makes me think of mean people who hate animals. Thunder makes me think people are going to hurt me. I want my food warm. I won't love Mom if my food isn't warm. Why aren't there any lizards now?"

"Because it's too cold," Laura and I say in chorus.

Tara begins an interesting dance of moving from her bed on Laura's right around the table counterclockwise to Laura's chair at the kitchen table to talk after Laura asks her a question. Then after Tara has communicated back, she goes behind Laura's chair to her bed again. She repeats this over and over with every conversation.

Tara continues, "Does the sun split in half? Laura is not human or animal. She is from a planet with two suns. You have a sun over your head and under your feet."

Laura asks me, "Do you know of a planet with two suns?"

"I'm not aware of this being possible according to the laws of physics, but what do I know?"

Laura asks Tara, "Do you like Cynthia and the fork tuning?"

"Cynthia isn't human either. She came from a star."

"How about your Mom?"

"She is from a big red desert rock—one that people go to pray."

"And what about you?"

"I am from a shooting star."

18

Dr. Uribe meets me at Cañada Larga at ten A.M. I put Genji's halter on and lead him out of his stall to the area for grooming and saddling for his barn. We talk briefly and when it begins to rain, we all go back into Genji's stall.

I explain that Genji told Laura that his pain goes from his left hip across his back and down the back of his right front leg. It also goes up his neck to his poll, or the top of his head, and that his jaw hurts when he goes downhill. Dr. Uribe, who I'm certain is completely skeptical of this "conversation," uses a small three inch long cylinder ball point pen looking instrument which he runs along Genji's sciatica nerves, neck and shoulders. This shows where the problems are which are indicated by twitching muscles, and an uncomfortable reaction to being touched. Amazingly enough it includes his left hip and sciatica, right shoulder, and right side of his neck.

Dr. Uribe manipulates his back, his hips, and his back legs. When he manipulates his front legs both ankles pop. When he works on the right side of his neck and shoulder—something pops in his left shoulder. I am standing in front of his head, so that I am able to see everything Dr. Uribe does.

"You have a fascinating career," I say in awe.

"I was a veterinarian for ten years before I studied this."

"You can learn something like this in this country?"

"I studied twenty years ago. Yes in this country." He doesn't say where.

Genji who is nervous and jumpy on a good day stands quietly, eyes shiny and deep while Dr. Uribe works on him. I had Laura prep him for this, so he would know what to expect. I guess that was a good idea.

After the chiropractic treatment is complete, Dr. Uribe says, "Okay now I am going to do acupuncture on him." He places needles along his back, but they are hollow. He then injects vitamin B-12 into each needle. He uses horse size hypodermic needles filled with a pink liquid.

"What does the B-12 do?"

"It goes into the blood and to the brain. The brain releases endorphins which alleviates his pain. He is in pain." He looks at me, "It's more complicated than that."

"This explanation is the short form?"

He laughs, "Yes. No hard exercise for two days. You can hand walk him. I should see him again in four weeks."

Dr. Uribe packs up his bag and walks to the stall next door to see his second patient. This is the mare that told Genji she thinks he is beautiful.

Now I understand Genji's reluctance to ride, and his complete unwillingness to go up hills. I feel inadequate about having taken six months to have a chiropractic veterinarian work on him. In all honesty, I didn't know about chiropractic veterinarians. It was a fellow boarder with a horse in the same barn who suggested it while we were both grooming our horses.

I thought something was wrong with Genji's feet. I wasn't far off target. It is his sciatic nerve going into his left hind leg, plus his shoulders and ankles. This all has to do with moving his feet. When I first moved him to Canada Larga and was trying to figure out what was wrong with him, I mentioned it to the manager, Natasha. She dismissed it as behavior, "He is being a butt-head."

Awful

When you've owned and ridden a horse for eleven years, you know the horse relatively well. This was not Genji's true attitude or behavior, and I felt summarily labeled as an incompetent know-nothing horse owner. People do this in all walks of life. If you aren't the authority with the degree to prove it, or the years of experience to vindicate it, well your intuition or instinct or knowledge doesn't count. I never thought Genji was being a "butt-head." I knew something was wrong. However, since his gait was smooth, and he didn't feel lame, I had only the refusal to go up a steep hill to go on. Also, he seems to tire easily, so our rides have been relatively short.

I am relieved that Genji is now on the road to recovery. And, I've learned that when I am convinced that something is not right with an animal, that the animal's action does not reflect what I know about the animal's behavior and attitude—well, something is wrong! I believe that the challenge then is to honor your conviction, and to explore ways to resolve the situation. I knew that I could not afford x-rays and surgery, so that was not an option. It is also apparent now that it would have been foolish to pursue that option. What does work is to listen to suggestions from others, and to filter out the ones that invalidate you. I add to my inventory of solutions to situations such as the animal communicator, the equine chiropractic veterinarian, the sound balancing. California is a fertile bed of alternative healing venues, and I find that exploring them is a journey into healing in unexpected ways. One of those unexpected ways has been for me to start taking the invalidation test. When I know down to my bones that I know my animal better than anyone else—then is someone's suggestion being constructive and contributing to helping me and my animal, or is it attitude, which invalidates the situation?

I ride Genji eight days after his treatment. I try to ride up two different canyons, but the heavy rains two weeks ago have eroded the trails severely. One is blocked by a huge oak tree that has fallen across it, and some of the edge of the trail has fallen off into the creek far below. Wild pigs have torn up the other side of the trail and the hillside above that. The mud is deep and riding is probably not safe. The second canyon is even muddier, so I turn back. I ride across green grass to a third canyon that is more in the sun and therefore drier. By now Genji is tiring. I also notice that he is having trouble walking on the rocks in the creek bed, and the slight incline going down into it is causing him to move his feet gingerly. Our ride is over—I head back to the barn wondering if we can ever really ride like we used to again. I realize that one treatment probably isn't going to solve his problem either.

It's a beautiful sunny day, but it does little to ease my heartache. My horse was abused and injured at his former stable. My dogs were abused at their own home. All of this while I thought they were being lovingly taken care of by others. I simply was too naïve to realize what was happening to any of them—dogs or horse. I didn't protect them. I didn't understand that people could be so mean or so insane. Only now that my life is evolved age-wise do I understand that one can never stop being vigilant. But it is more than being vigilant for me. I have lost trust in other people's abilities to be compassionate, to communicate honestly, or to care about the animals they are hired to look after. In a way it is very isolating.

I don't know what happened at the stable. I do know that whatever it was never happened at any other stable where Genji was boarded. In a stall now Genji is terrified when I walk behind him. I'm not certain he sleeps in his stall. It never looks used. If that is all that is wrong with him, I'd be happy. The physical damage he has suffered is possibly permanent, and in that case he is no longer a trail horse. He might be okay to ride in an arena, but for me that isn't riding, isn't fun, and not what I want to do.

I mentally commit to a series of six treatments before I give up and have to consider his possible retirement with all of the implications that includes. I am not moving him from "in front of Heaven's Gates," but a stall is an expensive habitat for a horse I can't ride. I agonize over all of the possibilities, and surrender myself to the unknown. I try to throw all of the what-ifs up to the sun on such a glorious day in an attempt to ease my burden of guilt over my negligence in supervising his care.

19

I decide to ride Genji only in the soft sand in the arenas. I don't want to injure him further, and if we are riding on a consistent surface, perhaps I can feel something that isn't obvious on the changing surfaces of a trail ride. I also decide to throw out the saddle pad on my English saddle, because it is old and could be causing discomfort. I ride with my second saddle, a modified McClellan, just to see if it makes a difference. The McClellan is a little like a western saddle with leather fenders and stirrups, but has no horn. It is lighter weight and cinches up differently. Once I'm in the saddle with its fleece pad in the saddle seat, I'm so comfortable, I'm wondering why I let this saddle be a tack room decoration for so many years.

On a Sunday, I have the large covered arena to myself. We walk around the perimeter once. I usually let Genji choose his speed. A flat walk is an unusual way for him to begin a ride. He is usually quite animated. So, I take note of this. We continue on with some laps in both directions in the corto, plus some one-hundred-eighty degree turns in the corners of the arena. Then I let him increase his speed to a largo. He seems to be trying to canter in his right front leg. I stop him, back him up—this is like rebooting a computer, and proceed forward. As we go down the long side of the arena he slows down to a walk, and then I feel it—his right front leg seems to buckle under him. Okay, that's it for today. We head back to his barn.

Later in the week on a Thursday when I go riding, there is a lesson in the covered arena, so I had for the polo field, which is fenced with a solid wood fence, and is presently used as a jumping course. This is much larger than the large covered arena, and is further away from the barns and other arenas. It is quiet with a generous view of the surrounding green hills. The coastal range is steep, the result of tectonic plates sliding beneath the ocean and a patchwork of fault lines which contribute to an amazing one centimeter of growth per year. The soil is loose with rocky outcroppings. The chaparral vegetation including chamise, scrub oak, mountain mahogany, white sage, and ceanothus, or California wild , lilac is drought hardy and is adapted to no moisture for six months a year.

We follow the same routine as our last ride. Genji chooses to walk with no sign of lameness. We ride at the corto around the arena multiple times. Then we try the largo—again an attempt to canter in his right front leg, slowing to a walk, and the buckling. That ends our ride, and finally I have two exact same physical situations to describe to Dr. Uribe when he comes tomorrow for Genji's second treatment.

"Good morning, Dr. Uribe, how are you?"

"How is Genji doing?"

It's hard for me to tell if his first treatment changed anything, but I didn't expect one treatment to solve his problem."

I explain everything that happened on our two previous rides. Genji likes Dr. Uribe. He stands still and receives the treatment as if it is a massage. After working on him for a while, Dr. Uribe feels something that has to do with Genji's right front leg. He pushes two long acupuncture needles into the back of Genji's heel. Genji flinches and tries to pull his foot away. The needles go in approximately three inches. They stay in his foot while Dr. Uribe works on his neck and puts more needles in his back.

"Do all of these points have names?"

"They all have names that are Chinese. We call the meridians by the names of the organ that it is associated with like liver or kidney. American vets usually call the points by numbers. People who use the Chinese names are more purist. I used to know all of the names, but that was twenty years ago, and now I use the numbers."

I move from Genji's right front to his left front to get out of Dr. Uribe's way. Dr. Uribe pulls Genji's head way around to his right side. Genji immediately picks his right front foot with the needles in it up high and stomps it down on the stall floor twice. I look at Genji. I look at Dr. Uribe, who has moved back, and I start to laugh. Dr. Uribe takes out the needles and is finished.

"You can ride Sunday. I'll see him in three to four weeks. He should be much improved after three treatments."

Today Dr. Uribe is treating four or five horses, all but one in Genji's barn. All of the horse owners in this barn are women. There are six stalls, six horses, six women. We share a tack room, and a saddling up area under a shady pepper tree. Since we seem to be there at overlapping times we talk, and friendships are growing.

20

"I feel like the oldest dog in the world."

"Rasa knocked Kundun down. He fell downhill in the yard and scraped his chin and nose."

"I'd rather have Rasa knock me down than knock myself down."

"I told him I'm sorry and if I could, I'd fix him a special meal—maybe Mom could make a beef stew for him?"

When Laura arrived I met her in the driveway. When she saw my short hair she made a comment about it.

In the kitchen, Kundun says, "I noticed her haircut and I wonder how many people do that?"

I laugh, "Not that many women get their hair cut one inch long."

"The issue today is that Tara goes berserk when the yard maintenance man is here Tuesday mornings. I have to put her in my office upstairs and close the door."

Laura talks to Tara, "There are calming things to do like licking your mouth, sniffing the ground, blinking your eyes, yawning, and looking away."

"What are you thinking, Kundun?"

"I'm thinking about peeing in the house. I'm not peeing for Mom. I drink less water."

"I pick up the water bowl at seven. Tara, the bump on the front of your neck is not a tumor. The vet did a biopsy on it, and it's some weird cluster of dried up white blood cells, maybe from a foxtail."

Tara is relieved, "I'm glad it's not cancer."

"How is my sister?" Rasa asks.

"She isn't pregnant yet."

"Does she know how to use a calculator? They are really complicated."

When I sit at the kitchen table, often I use a small calculator, and of course, Rasa watches everything I do. And as I've learned by now, dogs know more than they see or hear. Rasa and Tara get their dolls. Rasa gets her yellow ducky that quacks when she squeezes it between her teeth. Tara gets her very special purple fuzzy bear. They take their dollies to Laura. For them this is a huge love offering, especially for Tara.

Rasa has an ongoing concern about not seeing Genji, "He is forgetting me."

"The problem with Rasa going to the stable is that there is a pack of ranch dogs."

"Maybe I could stay in the car and Genji can come to the car."

"Well, that's an idea. I realize that I need to resolve this situation of the dogs and Genji missing each other."

"Do they have any questions for me?"

Kundun asks the first question, "Am I ever going back to the Big Land?"

I have a difficult time answering this for Kundun. He misses the ranch in New Mexico so much. He loves it there. As I grope for words, Laura tells him, "Mom is going in June, but you can never go back. It's too long of a drive. This is your life now."

Kundun graciously responds, "Okay, that's all right." He immediately changes the subject, "Does she think of me when she's buying something for the kitchen?"

"Like food?" I ask.

"A choppy thing."

Laura offers, "A food processor?"

"I never use one."

"It's hard to chew."

Laura lifts up his lip and we both look into his mouth. His gums are bright red and his back molars look infected. I'm shocked.

"Isn't it funny how he segues into a physical issue?" Laura observes.

"How fast do you read?" Rasa asks.

"I read medium fast. If I read too fast I skip words and have to re-read."

"You should read about dogs and old women on the prairie."

"How do you know about the prairie?"

"Kundun and I have been talking about how we miss the big open spaces."

"I miss it too. What did the two coyotes this morning say to you?"

Tara answers. "The coyotes said to stay away from them—one has a cough."

Rasa adds, "One coyote said I have the most beautiful eyes he's ever seen on any animal anywhere. They look like two moons."

Kundun says, "They said, 'Back off big guy! Have you seen any rabbits?'"

Kundun does not bark at Chatty, so these were two other coyotes including the coyote with the white tipped tail.

"It's time to say goodbye to Laura."

Laura stands up and Tara growls at her.

"I think she forgot who you are."

"I'm moving funny from my injury."

We get Tara to come close to Laura. "I forgot who you are."

This has started to happen with Tara. I always warn houseguests that they can come back downstairs and she will have forgotten who they are, and bark at them as if she'd never seen them before.

I make an appointment at Buena for Kundun in two days on Friday. Dr. Nicci looks at his gums and teeth. She decides that he needs his teeth cleaned plus a biopsy of his gum tissue. The appointment is scheduled in five days. This procedure entails Kundun having anesthesia, and the older my dogs become, the more fearful I am of general anesthesia.

However, Kundun does very well and when I arrive to pick him up in the afternoon, Dr. Nicci explains, "I had a difficult time getting a biopsy sample of his gum tissue because his gums are mushy."

When the biopsy results come back it is diagnosed as an immune disorder. His body has turned on itself. Dr. Nicci prescribes prednisone to counteract the gum issue.

During our next appointment with Cynthia, I update her on Kundun. She is an advocate for all natural healing and decides to investigate this. At our appointment following that one she hands me the results of her online investigation of metacam, the drug Kundun has been on for his arthritic pain.

"The metacam is causing Kundun's gum tissue problem. The immune disorder is one of the side effects. There is a website called metacamkills.com."

I am completely mortified to hear this and I immediately take him off the metacam. Kundun slowly recovers and regains his ability to eat kibble mixed with canned food. By now he has lost much more weight, but looks youthful and is happy.

21

"Genji, hello! It's so nice to see you again. Wow, you look beautiful!"

Laura is here for a visit. I give Genji an apple and put his halter on. We all walk over to a patch of grass by the small covered arena. Genji doesn't seem like he is communicating because he is busy eating the grass, but Laura has explained previously that she communicates with border collies while they are fetching balls.

"What do you want to communicate about today?"

"I want to know how Genji feels after having three treatments, how he feels while I'm riding, and if he's ready to try the hills yet."

"I feel a lot better, but there is still pain on top of my head that goes down my neck and into my left front leg. When we ride uphill it feels like my back is swayed down. So, I'm not ready to ride up steep hills. When we ride now Mom feels more free and not like she's trying to get me to perform."

"This started with his problems. Whatever he could do was what we did, and then we stopped. That was the ride." I laugh, "He still performs! He doesn't pull on the bit anymore and that makes a huge difference when we ride. Also he lets me put the bit in his mouth easily. He never has until recently."

"My mouth felt like it was pulled sideways because of all the lunging they did when I was younger."

"His legs look beautiful. Look at his legs! And his mane is so soft. He didn't look like this the last time I was here."

"I'm riding him twice a week. He is on new supplements now, and he does look wonderful doesn't he?"

"I need more supplements. I need double."

"I now use Smart Pak and they are pre-measured." Laura confers, and Genji wants more of the minerals and electrolytes. I am fairly amazed by how the animals will tell you what they need.

"I want what one of the horses behind me gets."

We figure out that it is not one of the horses in Genji's barn. It is a dark horse that ignores him that is in the barn behind him. The corrals in Genji's barn and the corrals in the large barn behind his barn face each other with a dirt road inbetween them. I decide to look into this.

"Tell us a story."

"The mean lady is mean during the day, but not at night. At night she comes over and says, 'Hello Genji' and talks to all of the horses."

My eyes get big and I whisper, "He means Natasha?"

Laura nods yes. We furtively look around us to make sure no one hears us.

"What do you mean by mean?" Laura asks.

"She says things to people that aren't nice."

"Genji is correct. I've heard it."

I'm really taken that animals observe everything. "Wow, and people think horses just stand around all day doing nothing!"

"Is there a foreman here?" Laura asks.

"Yes, Jose." I point to the man lunging a horse in the small covered arena.

"He has an ulcer from working for her."

"How do horses know things like that?"

"They either see a color where there is a problem, or see it in the person's mind."

"Tell us another story."

"The black and white dog got caught in some bushes (or a fence, or a fence and some bushes—this was not clear) and couldn't get out. The little brown dog ran to get Natasha to come help. She tried to get Natasha to follow her, but Natasha didn't understand. So the little brown dog got him out."

"We're hearing all of the gossip."

"Genji, Rasa and Kundun want to come visit, and Rasa thinks you are forgetting her."

"I am not forgetting the dogs, and in the night when I am bored, I come to visit them and we talk."

"Tell us a story you make up."

"Once upon a time there was a beautiful lady who had a beautiful horse. She built a nice barn for her horse, and every evening she came to the barn to say good night."

"I did that."

"He didn't make up that story?"

"No. I miss that too, Genji."

"Will I live at the house again?"

"Not where I am now. There is nowhere to build a barn and it's a steep hill. I'm thinking of finding a smaller house with more land so you can. I don't know what to do."

"Let's ask Genji what you should do," Laura suggests.

• "You are in the flow. You are not doing all of the things you want to do. Just stay where you are because I see that you are happy there. Do more of what you want to do, and just see what happens."

A Taoist guru in a cave at the top of a mountain couldn't have told me any wiser of words.

Then Genji talks to Laura, "I don't think you are happy doing what you are doing."

"You mean talking to animals?" She looks horrified.

"I mean on a larger scale."

"I'm working on that." Laura looks at me, "You don't write poetry do you?"

"Yes, I do, but not lately because I had a problem with line spacing on my computer, but I finally figured out how to fix it."

"Genji wants you to come out here and write poetry about horses and the valley."

"I'll do that, and put a chair in the stall to read him a book about horses. Remember, he asked me to do that."

When, I have no idea, but it's a goal. It's a goal to slow down, to try to dissolve the spin I'm in with errands, appointments and tiredness. The years creep by and I never take the time to do something completely radical like read a book to my horse.

It's time for Laura to leave. Genji returns to his stall for carrots and another apple.

"Bye bye Genji. I love you." I point at my eye, hold my right closed hand over my heart and then point at Genji—sign language for I love you.

22

Laura calls me in the evening to tell me that a woman has flown in from Santa Fe to do chiropractic work on some horses at my stable tomorrow, and would I want a treatment for Genji? I have planned a full office day and this does not fit into my schedule at all, but I decide not to pass up a treatment for him and a different opinion on his injury.

I arrive at Canada Larga at ten forty-five in the morning. I put Genji's halter on, and take him to the large barn behind his barn. Dr. Sherry is treating a horse in the aisle, standing on top of a mounting block to work on his back. She is diminutive and animated with the assurance of someone who has helped many horses. Dr Sherry is trained as an animal chiropractic. She treats cats, dogs and horses.

She asks a few questions, "When was Genji's injury?"

"One year ago. I'm not sure if this is something cumulative, or if one event caused his injury."

"How old is Genji?"

"He will be fifteen in May."

There is a swarm of women around Genji. There is the jumping trainer who is having several horses treated, and Laura's friend who is the contact person for Dr. Sherry. Genji is being fed cookies, Crystal is braiding his mane into an elaborate French braid along the top of his neck, and Genji seems to enjoy all of the attention. At his barn the women are all usually busy grooming, saddling up, and dashing off to the large covered arena for a lesson with their horses. Genji and I are the only ones in the barn who don't take lessons.

Dr. Sherry stands in front of Genji's head. "Come stand next to me and look at his head. Do you see how his left eye is lower that his right eye?"

I'm amazed. His left eye is indeed lower than his right eye. "I see that!"

"His head is tilted to one side. This means that his first vertebra is out of alignment." She steps around to the right side of his head and pulls on the top of his neck with her fingers. It looks like she is massaging his vertebra. She picks up his right front leg and bends it under him. She shows me how it doesn't have full mobility. She moves back to his right hip. When she barely touches it, he flinches.

"This hip is sore." She begins to massage his hip area, works on his back, lifts his tail to look at his posture, then moves to his left side. I follow along behind her trying to watch what she does. She picks up his left front leg and shows me how his hoof tips slightly sideways further demonstrating his misaligned body, plus how his leg does not bend with full mobility. She continues to work on him. He is fed cookies to divert his attention.

"He told Laura that his poll hurt, now I see why. He said that the pain went down his neck and crossed over his back diagonally to his hip, plus went down his front leg to behind his knee. These are all of the problem areas you are pointing out."

When Dr. Sherry massages his back his skin twitches and his muscles jump. She shows me how to massage his stomach to make his back rise up along his topline. "This is a good exercise for him to strengthen his back."

"Genji said that when he goes uphill his back feels swayed down. I think I understand that now."

"Don't pull on his poll. Don't let anyone touch it. If he is eating grass and you pull on the lead rope to get his head up, this pulls on his poll. Touch his nose with your foot instead."

"I never knew to do that."

"I just learned it myself." She bends each of his front legs and shows me how they now bend correctly.

At the end of the session we all hug and she gives me information about a non-invasive product for his skin cancer tumors.

"Walk him in a small circle each direction then a large circle each direction to let him feel his new body. Then give him a turn-out. It will take him four to six months to completely recover after this treatment."

I walk him in the circles then head for the turn-out arena. When I take off his halter he rolls and rolls. Instead of getting back on his feet right away like usual, he stays there with his front legs bent in front of him and his neck stretched out with his chin on the sand. I have never seen him do this. It looks like horse yoga. I watch him curiously wondering what he feels. He definitely has to feel better. Then he rubs his cheeks and face on his knees, and gets back up. He likes to sniff the sand to see who has been in the arena. While he does this he keeps his nose near the ground while moving along in his corto gait. This always amuses me. He comes past me where I am standing in two square feet of shade next to the fence. He spins and gallops making quick turns and sudden sand throwing stops. He snorts then spins away in a gallop continuing to go back and forth in front of me. I think this is the smoothest, most fluid he has looked while galloping around in a turn-out and I am very happy. When he is finished he comes over so I can put the halter on. We walk back to his barn.

23

I make the mistake of scheduling an appointment with Laura on the morning my landscape maintenance man comes to work. The courtyard off the kitchen is part of the outside dog area, and is visible through the glass doors. I chase Kevin out with his leaf blower and garden tools, all of which send Tara into a crazed frenzy. Normally I keep her in my office upstairs with the door closed until he leaves.

Laura sits down and looks at Tara, "How are you feeling?"

"Barking works me up and gives me an adrenaline rush, which gives me a headache. I feel good in my body. I like my food. My right elbow and shoulder hurt and it goes into my foot."

"How are you feeling, Rasa?"

"I feel better in my body than I have for a long time. My teeth feel better, and I won't go back there again!"

"You have to go back one more time to get your teeth finished," I respond.

"No! It's my choice and I won't go!"

Poor Rasa. I left her and Tara at a kennel while I drove north on a business trip to the bay area. It was a relatively short time - a weekend plus the drive both directions. I had left them at this kennel one previous time, and it seemed like everything had been okay, although I didn't like the evasive response to my question inquiring how they had been while there. At the conclusion of the event my plan was to spend the night at the hotel and leave early in the morning. As I arrived back at my room my intuition blasted me with "leave now!" I immediately packed up, checked out, and began the drive home. Because it was mid-afternoon when I left Pleasanton, I spent the night in Paso Robles. I drove straight to the kennel unannounced one day earlier than expected. Again there were evasive answers to my questions concerning their well-being.

That night Tara threw up on the bed. We made the run to the kitchen door, and while she was outside I ran back upstairs to clean up the mess. Once I had my glasses on I could see that she had thrown up multiple pieces of spongy foam. In the morning I found more pieces that she had thrown up outside. In all Tara threw up some twenty-five pieces of spongy foam over a twenty-four hour period. I got nowhere with a phone call to the kennel.

What I didn't realize until Dr. Nicci looked into her mouth after I had noticed a broken tooth was that Rasa had multiple broken and fractured teeth from being at that kennel. Dr. Nicci sent us to a canine dental surgeon in Ventura. Her main client is the Ventura County Sheriff's Department K-9 unit. Large photographs of toothy German Shepherds and their macho deputy handlers cover the walls of the clinic. Rasa had to have three incisors and one canine removed as well as have two root canals to preserve a molar and a canine. The second appointment is to complete the root canals.

I can't imagine what kind of frenzy Rasa and Tara were pushed into that caused Tara to rip up and eat her bed, and Rasa to chew on the chain link fence in an attempt to escape. They would never go there again. We interviewed at Kay's, and although Rasa and Tara need to be kept separate from the other dogs, thankfully Kay was willing to board them anyway.

"What do you think of Kay's, Rasa?"

"There are dogs there crazier than Tara!" To me Rasa instructs, "You have to write what's on your mind. You have to work-out your mind."

Rasa is my coach and always gives me things to ponder or do. She intently watches me write in the mornings.

Kundun enters the conversation, "Don't put me on canned, it gives me diarrhea. I like the raw food. What I'm eating now makes my heart work right. Will we sleep together at Kay's?"

Laura explains the sleeping situation to me, "The dogs sleep in cubicles." To Kundun, "You'll sleep alone."

"You know what I like about it there? The girls keep telling me how cool I look," Rasa adds.

Tara changes the subject dramatically, "It feels like this hill is going to slide down. There's an underground river here."

I look at Laura, "Does she mean there is an underground river here, or an underground river at the ranch, because there is supposedly one there."

"No, the river is here."

"Are you going somewhere special?" Tara inquires.

And again, I am confronted with having to let them know that I am going to Santa Fe, the ranch, the big land, and that they aren't coming with me, that we aren't going to ever live there again. "We're all too old. We can't go up and down the mountains any more—not me, not Genji, not you dogs."

Kundun offers, "Can't we all live there without going up the mountains? If you sell the big land then we'll all be homeless."

Laura states emphatically, "No, you have this place. This is your home now."

"We'll be homeless in our dreams," Kundun laments.

"I feel like I said goodbye when I left," Tara says.

"I say goodbye to the healthy animals there. The animals there feel much healthier than here," Rasa adds.

"Why aren't they as healthy here?" I venture.

"They have a different kind of smell, it smells toxic. They don't see as well."

"Where are the coyotes?" I'm curious because I haven't seen or heard them for the past month.

"There is a man shooting them, and they moved to where the house is being built. They are eating garbage the workmen leave."

"Do you have any questions for me?"

"How long will you be gone?" Tara asks.

"Seventeen days." Laura has explained to me that she communicates a day by showing one day and one night. She seems to be able to do this quickly. I try to do this if it is a few days, but I switch into the moon phases for a longer period of time.

"Are you bringing anything back from the ranch?"

"Do you want me to bring back something?"

Laura receives Tara's image, but is completely stumped by it, "It looks like she is showing me large metal and glass candlesticks with fire coming out of the top, and also a large book."

I point at the glass candlesticks on the kitchen table, "These are what I had on the table there." I mentally scan the great room in the house at the ranch the way it looked when we lived there. "Oh, she means the iron dragon andirons in the fireplace! They are right here in this fireplace, but I never use the fireplace because it doesn't work, so she doesn't know they are here. Also I boarded the dogs at a kennel while the movers were there. They never saw the house empty. I picked them up and we drove to California."

As for the large book, I realize later that it is my National Geographic World Atlas, which I used to look at frequently, but not since we moved. I am both stunned and fascinated by what Tara remembers and has noticed missing in our lives, and more than that—what she perceives as needing to be included as it once was for a sense of balance. My SofA |CHARM

Tara then asks, "Are you happier here or there?"

"I'm healthier here. I can breathe better." I sidestep the happiness answer.

"Maybe you should write a poem and hide it in the wall there."

I love Tara's idea! "I'll do that and it will be about you."

"Do you have a question, Kundun?"

"Did you tell Genji you are going, and is someone going to give him his medications?"

"Yes, I told him, and someone will give him his supplements."

"Okay Rasa, your turn."

"What are you going to do when someone gets angry at you?"

"I'm not aware that someone is going to get angry at me."

"Some people just want money from you."

"How do you know that?"

"I see motivations in the air. We will be fine at Kay's. You can take your trip, relax and not worry about us."

24

I am driving from Ojai to Santa Fe to attend my grandson's sixth grade graduation from Desert Montessori School where he has attended school since pre-school. I like to drive no more than six to seven hours, so for me it is a several day drive. I enjoy looking at the scenery and thinking as I wend my way through the landscape. Rasa and Tara have traveled thousands of miles with me—this route seven times. All along the way I recall where we stayed, where I went to dinner or lunch, where we stopped for little walks and potty breaks.

Tara, who has a tendency to get motion sickness, gets a Bonine, and sits in the single back seat. It is outfitted with an Orvis seat cover and a folded cotton patchwork quilt with different breeds of dogs on it. She watches the scenery and seldom lies down unless I have stopped to eat. The double seat next to her is folded up against the back of the driver's seat and the console space in between the front seats. Rasa has an Orvis bed especially made for the rear end of SUV's, which is covered with a second same patterned dog quilt. She shares this space with my luggage and the dog baggage, which is the equivalent of traveling with two small children. There are two flannel sheets for putting on the hotel beds because they sleep on the bed with me. There are towels to place on any sofas because they lie on those. They have their own bag with dishes, supplements, and some of their food. Because I've learned that I can't find their food just anywhere—there is all of the kibble and canned food they will need for the entire time we are gone. There is a gallon plastic container of filtered water from home because if I won't drink tap water anywhere—they aren't either. I refill it along the way with purchased water.

We've enjoyed our trips together, and I've loved their company while I drive. This time though I'm feeling sad knowing we are running out of time. I'm scared to lose my dogs. Okay, stay in the present I admonish myself. It's not just my dog's lives that have flown by—it's my life as well.

I stay at La Posada in Winslow, Arizona my second night after a pleasant drive through the Mojave desert with surprisingly low temperatures in the sixties and low seventies. Needles is the hottest at eighty-two degrees. La Posada is a huge rambling former Fred Harvey Hotel that sits next to the railroad tracks. It was designed by Mary Coulter and inspired by the great haciendas of the Southwest. I stay in the Howard Hughes Suite with a giant carved wood four-poster bed. Windows look into gardens below. I dine in the Turquoise Room gourmet restaurant, one of the ten best restaurants in Arizona. I think that one of my favorite things to do when I travel is to stay in a remote-seeming hotel that is almost out of context with where it is—being elegant and serving gourmet food. La Posada is very popular. The parking lot is full and rooms are booked months in advance. The dining room is busy, and each table has a view of the trains going by the windows.

Dining car memorabilia are sold in the dining room area. Authentic dining car serving dishes, sugar bowls, cream pitchers and silverware are displayed in cases in the lobby. I remember all of those from the train rides I took with my grandparents in the 1940's. It doesn't seem that long ago that my sister and I took the train trips with our grandparents. Now we are the grandparents.

When visiting my son's home in Santa Fe, I find myself alone in the kitchen as I perch on a stool at the island counter. Bhakti comes to me looking much older and ravaged by the attack on him several months earlier. We look into each other's eyes, "Bhakti, we moved far away from here. That's why you don't see Rasa, Tara and Kundun anymore. That's why there aren't any more barbeques at the ranch. I'm saying goodbye to you from all of us because we won't see you again. Don't give up Bhakti—Alan needs you to look after him. I love you Bhakti. We all love you. We miss you."

I don't know if Bhakti understands me—I hope so. He is rarely still, but while I am trying to communicate with imagery he is very still and attentive, his light amber eyes deep and expressive. He is a beautiful boy with a big, fun heart. I think of him jumping back and forth across the creek as Will commands him, "Over, over, over." He never seemed to tire as a young dog. He is slipping away now—twelve years old, going on thirteen. I reflect on the meaning of his name, Bhakti—devotion.

While in Santa Fe I visit my land several times. Because of heavy winter snows and spring rain, it is green and lush. Both creeks are flowing, even the Ojo Sarco, which has been dry for years due to drought, and the suspicious results of a real estate development drilling a well next to the creek bed higher up the valley. My daughter, who is also in Santa Fe for the graduation, and I hike up to the pool and waterfall that are on land formerly owned by her. We are elated to see the waterfall flowing over the thirty foot cliff into a filled crystal clear pool below. It has been at least seven or eight years since there has been water here other than flash floods. I wonder if the salamander survived after all of that time. I remember jumping into the pool naked, and screaming because the water is freezing. But it felt good on a hot day, so I did it every summer repeatedly.

While I walk where Rasa, Tara, Kundun and I used to walk, I could hear them—Tara baying and chasing a rabbit, Rasa cutting a straight line through Tara's circles, and Kundun just running because he was so excited, and had no idea that Rasa and Tara were executing a hunting tactic. In California they talk about returning to the big land. And here I am back at the big land without them.

As I sit at the Sacred Pool, I contemplate their questions for me before I left home. "We can't come back and not go up the mountains, Kundun. The mountains are the place and they are steep in this little canyon. Just the short hikes I have taken to the waterfall and pool, and the cave are a challenge for me. We are all getting older now. To think that I designed and built all of these miles of trails, and then maintained them, and hiked on them all of the time—now it takes a lot of effort and I go slowly. No, Kundun, those days belong to our youth, and our younger, more physical and energetic days. They are a memory now. With your arthritis, you would have a difficult time here. We had to say goodbye to our rugged, isolated little canyon. It will always be a special place in our hearts, Kundun, and don't worry—you will never be homeless in your dreams. The spirits all protect it and welcome you to run and play here. The land belongs to the spirits. People are only passers-by in a continuum we can barely grasp. Just think about those petrified logs in Bear Hollow.

"I am happier in California, Tara. It's easier with my asthma to live at sea level. We aren't thirty-five miles from a grocery store or restaurant now. We don't live on a four-wheel drive road anymore. I know that you miss the wild crazy runs through the ponderosas and pinons, splashing across the creek, and jumping in the pools for a cool dip. I miss all of that too, Tara—the hikes, the rides on Genji—you and Rasa always with me. But I had a fear while we were covering miles of National Forest. I feared that you or Rasa would get shot by one of the local crazies out for sport. That's why we avoided the roads. After we moved, Karla's dog, Jasmine, did get shot. Mark, who was taking care of the place after we moved, found her in a pile of dead dogs on one of his exploratory hikes. He found a trap line also, with coyotes and foxes in it. So, it is open, wild, and wonderful here, but it is dangerous as well. I worried about you every time I let you out the door to take a hike, Tara, because you would race off baying and barking. At the end of a hike I'd return to the house, but that didn't mean you would until you were ready to. That's why we always hiked in the early afternoons and I fed you dinner after we got back. Now, after your embolism, you can't run like that. Your little legs shake when we take the smallest of walks. So, Miss Tara, instead of living on the big land, we live in the big house sharing all of those memories as we gather in the kitchen.

"Your question, Rasa, is the most difficult to answer. Nature just is. There is no nonsense, no deception. A terrific thunder and hail storm can instantly release a cascade of brown churning water down every hillside funneling it into every arroyo until a flood is roaring and sweeping through the canyon carrying fallen trees, boulders, and everything in its way. This in turn rips out fences, bridges, the road, and then when it slowly subsides there is forest debris left behind like children's toys. It happens. It is phenomenal to witness, and when it's over the sun comes out. Piles of hail look incongruent in the green of summer. You accept it for what it is.

"I learned, Rasa, that nature is true to itself, is real, and unbearably honest. People, though, have a tendency to try to control, manipulate, and when reality isn't the perfection they expect or want, then they can become out of control emotionally. Your question is about anger specifically. Yes, anger is very destructive. It can ruin relationships of all kinds. I've experienced both: the outward vicious expression of it, or the more subtle, insidious aspect of abusing the dog, which is what happened to poor Tara. So, what am I going to do when someone gets angry at me? I'm walking away from it, Rasa. I don't want it in my life. I think that's the honest thing to do. After every storm in the canyon winter or summer—the sun always came out. Bright, brilliant sun dazzling everything in its light. I want to remember that, Rasa, because walking away is not engaging in it, is feeling the sunshine no matter what destruction just occurred."

Before I drive out I wander around my little log house looking for a place to hide the poem that I brought with me as Tara suggested. After unsuccessfully trying to stick it somewhere in the massive rock fireplace and chimney, I decide on a crack in a log. I feel like I am on a secret mission. I read it one last time.

TARA'S POEM

They are both running, hunting fools
Wild yelp filled chase after a rabbit
race toward turkeys
vanishing with a flap of giant wings
Bear surprised up a ponderosa
tough these girls
would have confronted a cougar

Those joyful days gone
Rasa fights cancer
surgery and chemo sucking her vitality
Tara collapsed in a helpless whimper
some strange embolism in her back
She walks unsteadily on a leash

Now we nurse our aging bodies in the kitchen
keep each other company
gather together our memories
Wonder how ten years disappeared
in a blur of happy abandon
The high country just a dream now.

Then I fold it up, and with a conspiratorial smile, "Okay Tara, I hid it!"

25

Within one week of my arriving home Kundun begins to refuse all food. I observe him passing black poop. Other than that, and lying on his bed looking miserable, there are no symptoms. I begin to give him some stomach and intestinal issue medications left from Rasa and Tara. He refuses everything.

No! Call vet ASAP!

Meanwhile I have a scheduled gum graft appointment with my periodontics dentist following the July Fourth weekend. On top of a sick dog and mouth pain, I have several unexpected houseguests. I have an overnight visit from a young granddaughter-like friend who is at San Diego State University. We have a wonderful visit. I have known her since the day she was born. On the weekend Cassidy comes from LA for lunch, and my sister comes to visit for two days.

On the weekend after Kundun does finally eat a little canned food mixed with rice, he vomits in the night. It is brownish black with dark blood in it. As soon as Buena opens I make an appointment. On Monday, I take my sister to visit Genji. She hasn't seen him for years. I have recently been working on my estate planning, and I have asked her to take care of him if anything happens to me and I can no longer care for him. She has a beautiful horse property in northern California where she raises Lusitanos for dressage. Lusitanos are descended from Andalusians and primarily found in Portugal and Brazil.

After a visit to the stable, Kundun, who came with us, goes to Buena. Dr. Jan who usually has a happy smile and engaging dark eyes framed by short dark hair sees him, and I've never seen her look so concerned. He doesn't even have his temperature taken. Based on what I have observed, and that he is dehydrated, Kundun is ushered out of the room to get an IV immediately. I sign the paperwork agreeing to the procedures and the cost—fifteen hundred dollars.

I just paid twelve hundred dollars for my dental work, and Rasa's appointment for her second and final dental surgery to complete the root canals is four days away. I received a letter from my Mastercard stating that I had gone over my limit—Rasa's first dental surgery for almost three thousand dollars—and that every charge from now on for an indefinite period of time will be charged thirty percent interest. So, obviously this credit card needs to be paid off and retired. I've used my master card for two years to pay the vet bills, almost exclusively. I've never been able to get it under five figures, so now I have no choice. I cut it up and plan to try to pay it off.

It never occurred to me to get health insurance for my dogs when they were puppies. I never thought of the ramifications of having three senior dogs simultaneously ten years down the road. I have no reference for my own aging process since my parents died at relatively young ages, and my two grandmothers still lived at home then died suddenly. As I've cared for my dogs, I have gained much insight into my own possible future situation. I have recently applied for long term care health insurance. I have updated my estate planning including my right to die in a living will. I believe that one should think about dying, because we will die, just as our pets will die.

Kundun is diagnosed with possible bleeding ulcers and comes home at the end of five days. He can stay home if he takes his medications and eats without any problems. Because I tried to <u>force medications</u> down his throat <u>before taking him to the vet,</u> he thought he was being abused, an apparent flashback to puppyhood. At home before I did this, he simply took all of his medications in little cream goat cheese balls. At Buena his medications were accomplished with hypodermic needles. Buena sends him home with a case of canned food for digestive issues, and multiple prescriptions that I am told to roll into the food like little meatballs—but don't let him see me do it!

The first problem is that the food doesn't roll into little meatballs, it disintegrates. After I attempt to do this for six different shapes and sizes of pills, I have to wash my hands with a brush to get the dog food out from under my fingernails. After all of this effort, Kundun gently picks through all of the food leaving pills exposed, then simply walks away. I try this three times. Nothing changes. I decide to try the cheese balls with him again.

Dr. Nicci calls, "I don't think Kundun has ulcers. This is a reaction to the prednisone he has been taking for his gum issue. Discontinue giving him the prednisone."

Kundun thankfully eats the cheese balls with the pills inside, and slowly begins to improve. He doesn't like the veterinarian clinic issued food, so I return the unopened cans and put him back on his former canned food. Kundun's

[handwritten marginal note:] WHY WOULD YOU DO this?

fragile state has turned our family up-side-down. I never leave for more than three hours. Kundun is no longer comfortable staying outside, so when I leave I make sure he has a walk to the oak grove for a potty break, and leave him in the kitchen. I give him extra pats and rubs and encouraging words continuously. I spend more time in the kitchen with my pack.

26

Laura arrives and sits in the kitchen. "How are you, Kundun?"

"My stomach feels like it has a ring of jingling keys in it. I think I have a made up disease and I want to stop taking all pills. I didn't like not being able to get treats at the hospital."

Rasa has an idea, "Mom should tie magnets to him and not take them off until he's better."

"Why?"

"His energy is all screwed up. He needs to get better or he's going to get a urinary tract infection." To Kundun, "I'm only telling you this because I love you."

Kundun states to no one in particular, "Thank you for saving my life."

Laura asks Rasa, "Can you hear okay?"

"I can hear better than Kundun."

"I can hear an owl far away," Kundun responds.

"There is an issue with anesthesia causing deafness in some of my clients."

In the early mornings Rasa and Tara sniff around the fountain outside the kitchen then follow a scent to an oak tree where they jump and bark. "What are you barking at in the tree? I've looked and looked, but I can't figure it out."

"Rats times two with babies in their pocket," Rasa blurts out.

I am taken with the math and the image. "Could it be opossums?"

"I think it's a rat—it runs fast," Tara adds.

Laura turns toward Tara in her bed, "What are you thinking?"

"The bed is uneven like it's rumpled."

Laura and I discuss all of the beds. "Is it one of the beds here in the kitchen? It can't be the one in my office—that's new."

"She's showing me a light bed and only you and she are on the bed."

"I am obsessive about bedding not being rumpled."

"Tara noticed that it hurt when Rasa and Kundun were gone."

"That is when Kundun was staying at the vet, and Rasa stayed in the kitchen the night of her second dental surgery, because she was still coming out of the anesthesia. Tara was very upset while Kundun was gone."

"Don't take me to the doctors. They don't know it, but I don't like them," Tara adds.

Laura recommends taking Tara to see Steve Matzkin, "I send lots of dogs to him even though he is a human chiropractor."

Kundun dramatically changes the subject, "When you die, do you die easy or hard?"

"Everybody dies differently," Laura answers.

"I never thought I'd die, but I'm glad you saved my life."

Tara has something else on her mind, "Mom needs places to walk—a place with shrines to pray, and we all make offerings." Dogs picking up Mom's upset

I'm fairly amazed by this, because I had shrines everywhere on the big land, and who would think dogs would notice especially hounds busy chasing rabbits and squirrels. I'm particularly touched by, "we all make offerings." I'm beginning to realize that we didn't just move and leave a place. We changed our way of being in the process, and that is now what I am beginning to understand that Tara, Rasa, Kundun, and Genji all miss so deeply.

We discuss where to do this, and decide on the front area below the house. "Have it facing the house not the road. I want an animal shrine." Tara instructs.

I visualize the animal shrine next to the Oriental Hotel in Bangkok beneath a gigantic spreading banyan tree. There are dozens of elephants, tigers, and assorted other animals made of clay, plastic and ceramic. I think this is what Tara means. I love her idea.

Tara is talkative today. "When Laura comes, I can feel your animals and they are wondering when you will come home. Sometimes your white cat comes here and wanders around."

This sounds very mysterious, and Laura explains, "There is training for psychic spies which includes mind travel and out-of-body experiences. My cat loves it, but I don't like it."

"Bhakti looks very old, and I told him goodbye from all of us. He had a terrible accident in March. He got out of the house unnoticed and something severely attacked him. I wonder if it was a wild animal, but William is certain it was a dog, or dogs. His neck was slashed up to his back. His nose and jaw were crushed and he lost all of his teeth because of that."

"Why didn't they euthanize him?" Laura asks.

"That is what I wondered."

Rasa and Kundun explain, "Bhakti is holding the family together."

"You know how people have hurt me? People have hurt Bhakti too," Tara adds.

"Cassidy loves you very much. You've been a good mom to all of us and to her. We love you," Rasa states.

This ends our conversation. There are so many questions. Does Bhakti think he is holding the family together or is he really holding it together? Do animals perceive reality from their point of view or from a universal point of view? Laura believes that the animals speak the absolute truth.

I hear, they are directly connected to Source

27

It is a quiet, sunny morning at the stable on Friday. When I drive in, I am surprised to see few cars and no riders. I take Genji out of his stall and begin to brush him as we wait for Laura.

She arrives and joins us, "Hello Genji, wow, you look beautiful! He looks like he's gained weight. He looks incredible."

"He is now getting the supplement that the Lusitano stallion gets—Platinum Performance, and he'll start the same grain next week."

After Genji has said, "I want what the dark horse with the dark spots on its face that ignores me eats," I walk along the six corrals at the large barn that face his corral. I look closely at each horse. I do this several times on different days, because there are three dark horses. It is the dark spots on the face description that challenges me. I finally decide that the horse on the end which does have faintly darker colors of brown on his cheeks must be the horse Genji means. I know who owns the horse in the corral next to him, so weeks later when I am there when the owner happens to be walking that horse, a dapple Lusitano gelding, I ask her if she knows what the horse next to hers eats. He is also her horse she tells me, so I tell her the story of how Genji has requested to eat what he eats. We laugh.

"I have Genji on a supplement for promoting gastric health, one for preventing parasites and worms, one for weight gain, plus the ones he has been on for healthy hooves, electrolytes, and a calming supplement."

"What do you have to tell us, Genji?"

"There are raccoons here at night. They try to eat our food, but we don't let them. I have more energy now than every horse here."

"Even the young horses?"

"The moms of the young horses don't care about them as much as mine does."

Laura and I are standing very close to Genji's head. His dark eyes gather us in from under his thick, long, black, gray, and white forelock. He stands very still while we are talking beneath the pepper tree in front of his barn. There are no distractions anywhere today.

Genji asks, "Can we ride over the top of the mountain?"

I look up at the power line tower on top of the hill above us and point with my chin, "We rode up there last week and it was a tough ride. It is all up getting there and all down getting back, no trees, no shade. I thought I'd killed him."

"There is a lake somewhere. Let's go there," Genji suggests.

"If you ride from the tower further up and go through a gate, you can see the ocean, does he mean that?"

Laura and Genji confer. "No, there is a lake." Genji is always giving me a quest!

"We rode on the new trail twice, then a bull escaped from an adjoining property and now the gate is closed, but I can't figure out how to open it. Genji wouldn't stand still and I was worried that he would bump into the barbwire."

"They have been talking about that gate. There is something you have to slip over to open it," Genji explains.

"You have to stand still so Mom can figure out what to do and open it," Laura says to Genji.

I visualize the chain around the tree and the odd section of chain around the gate, which is barbwire, and fairly unmanageable with a jumpy, nervous horse that wants to get going on the ride. There is a large round link on the end, and although that looks attached to the chain around the tree it must come off somehow.

"I want to do something different."

"You don't want to move to a new stable do you?"

"No I want to learn something new."

"I'll read to you."

"I want you to write what we talk about and read it to me."

"Genji, how do you like your mane braided like this? It looks so good," Laura asks.

I have been French-braiding his mane to keep it from tangling. His mane hangs down below his shoulder, so it is long and braids easily. The braid is done by bringing in mane from one side, so it is like a sideways French braid that ends near his withers.

"The other horses say I look like a mare."

Laura and I both laugh.

"Horses love to tease each other," Laura adds.

"I want a miniature horse," Genji states.

Laura confers with him, and explains, "He means a foal." She then realizes that Genji has somehow been with her when she has talked to two different horse clients. One of them is a mare with a foal. Looking absolutely amazed, Laura asks, "How do you do that?"

"The dogs miss you, Genji. It's so hard to bring them here with the ranch pack marauding everywhere."

"I am tired of them barking all night long. One of them ate a squirrel in front of me! Do you eat meat?"

"Yes," I say tentatively.

"Horse meat?"

"No!"

"Is Tara okay?"

"I think she is doing okay."

"She seems sad."

"She is in her bed a lot, but she is playful before dinnertime."

"I think she is sad because she is losing her senses."

"She stepped in a gopher hole on our evening walk below the house a few days ago so I have to be more careful even though I have her on a leash. She doesn't hear me call her unless I am in the same room."

"Can you build a barn at the house so I can live there?"

I look at Laura. I look at Genji who so wants to live where I live like how it used to be at the ranch in New Mexico. "There isn't room to build a barn at my house. There is nowhere to ride. I will try to solve this problem. For now you are here."

My heart aches every time he brings this up. Genji wants to live at home. The dogs miss the big land. Had I known, I would have focused on looking at completely different properties. I did look at facilities for horses. The houses were million dollar tear-downs with no access to trails. I'm not sure this will ever be resolved.

During the night I wake up and remember the dream I had last week. A young, very attractive man is with me. He says, "I wish I could live with you." I realize now that it had to have been Genji coming to me in human form. So, I send Genji a dream: A beautiful cremello mare that sparkles in the moonlight with a flowing white mane and tail and blue eyes quietly walks up to his stall. She magically unhooks the stall door with her lips, pushes the gate-like door open, and with a mischievous snort invites Genji to join her on a gallop through grassy meadows, sturdy hooves scattering moonlight all the way to the ocean where they stand in the dunes gazing into the quiet, mysterious fog. Waves lap the shore below them.

28

I arrive at Steve's with Rasa and Tara. His directions are the treasure hunt kind: "I'm on Tico Road. The driveway is across from the feed store. Go all the way down the driveway to the gate and honk—I'll let you in."

Hens and roosters scatter, small dogs bark, a collection of Harley Davidson motorcycles is parked in front of a RV. Large trees shade the area except in the only place there is to park. I leave the air conditioning on in the car and get out with one thought, "How am I going to get Rasa and Tara through this obstacle course of critters to chase!" This must look like a party to the hounds. A shirtless man with a wild gray mane appears.

"Are you Steve?"

"No." He disappears then reappears buttoning a Hawaiian shirt. "Just kidding, I'm Steve."

He ushers us past the motorcycles and into his chiropractic studio. We talk briefly about Rasa and Tara. He is befriending them as he feels their backs. The dogs think this is a love fest, especially Rasa. Tara is more interested in smelling all of the strange looking equipment that chiropractors have in their offices. Rasa has two vertebrae out of place, her fourth lumbar and atlas. He gets her to stand straight and pushes down on each vertebra separately.

"I adjust anything with vertebrae. I had a guy bring me his ducks to adjust. I adjusted a fish once. It was floating upside down."

"I thought that means they are dying."

"I think it lived a little longer."

Tara has a thoracic vertebra adjustment.

"This may change their behavior. If a dog has been in pain, it makes the dog grumpy. Call me in two days and let me know how they are doing."

Rasa and Tara do nothing but sleep for a week. Rasa still has the funny little movement in her front legs. Steve said that he had only ever seen one other dog walk like that and he thought it was genetic. What does happen is that Rasa becomes more animated, playful, and silly like she was before the cancer. She seems to have more energy. Tara is more playful and silly when it is dinner time. For the first time in two years I feel a thread of normal moving through each day.

Kundun seems to have recovered from his intestinal issues. He lost so much weight that he looks like he did eight years ago as a three year old. Because he is now off all of the drugs, he moves very stiffly with a little old man shuffle. Cynthia has him on Chinese herbs in a pill called "Mobility." Kundun's attitude as always is happy with a big grin to prove it. While he was hospitalized, I was surprised that Tara was so upset and depressed. Yes, he did almost die, but I didn't realize their closeness.

Two months pass with no emergency trips to the vet, no illnesses, no huge vet bills. It feels like a miracle after two years of non-stop drama and expenses. We have some equilibrium now. The days grow shorter and the nights cooler. Shadows lengthen as equinox spirals closer. The poison oak turns ruby red and reminds me of the Virginia creeper in New Mexico which always turns red first. Topaz leaves shimmer on locust trees making me think of the box elder maples along the creek on the big land.

With cooler days as well, I make an effort to get the dogs out of the house for a stimulating change of scenery. Rasa and Tara come to the stable. I back the car under the pepper tree at the east end of the parking area so they can lie in the back of the car and stay cool. I take Genji to the car to say, "Hello." I also take Rasa and Tara to Krotona, a theosophical center, for walks. I love their sign, "Dogs, keep your humans on a leash!" Also, the excellent bookstore always has treats for dogs, and they are allowed to go inside. Kundun goes to the stable as well, but I am able to let him out of the car because he is sociable with the ranch dogs.

I begin to do stretching exercises at home. At first I am in so much pain from the most minimal movements, I can't believe it. I keep doing them. I don't know if I feel better or not. My lower back hurts all of the time, yet there was a time when it didn't. I had a regular routine of stretching and working out at the gym. I keep hearing Rasa telling me to stretch—it will make me feel better. I am slowly able to bend further and reach farther. I add more stretches and one day I realize that I am not in pain, nor in pain hours later, or even at night when I wake up. Rasa is right!

I cringe when I see Tara run for the kitchen door to come in, but stumble on the two cobblestone steps on the way. I don't know if this is nerve damage from her embolism, or because her vision is failing. She doesn't hear me call her from twenty feet away. I don't want to be loud, so I move closer and clap my hands. She hears that. She spends most of her time in her bed in the kitchen. She doesn't join me in my office anymore, or come tell me it's her dinnertime by running into the office and flinging herself onto the oriental rug and rolling onto her back so that I will get out of my chair and rub her tummy. She doesn't spend hours outside like she used to. She lies in her bed sad eyes watching the days go by. I think of Genji's words, "I think she is sad because she is losing her senses."

I make a point of being happy for the dogs, of being affectionate with each of them, of making everything special, because I have no idea how long we will be together from now on. Losing them—each of them, all of them—will be extremely heartbreaking whenever it is. I try to live in each moment, laugh at myself, and to say, "I love you" to Genji, Kundun, Rasa and Tara every day. They are my best teachers, my special friends. The rest of our journey together unfolds one day at a time.

29

At night when Rasa and Tara are on the bed, I give them each a little massage. I am feeling for lumps or anything new and unusual on their bodies. They love the attention and have no idea about my covert intentions. During this process I feel a hard lump next to Tara's vertebrae in her mid-back. Every night I check it, and suddenly it is much larger, somewhat asymmetrical, and very hard. *VET - WHY NO CALL*

! If I have learned one thing in the past two years, it is to act quickly. I take Tara to Buena to see Dr. Jill who is available on Tuesday morning. Dr. Jill, like Dr. Jan, is from Hawaii. She is youthful with dark hair, dark eyes, and is enthusiastic about being a veterinarian. Dr. Jill gives Tara an exam plus aspirates the lump for a quick look under the microscope. The lump is difficult to get a sample from, and therefore is suspicious.

"There are some long spindly cells and I think we should get a biopsy. Tara is so upset by any procedure that she will need a general anesthesia for the biopsy."

I make a quick decision, "I want the lump removed and the biopsy done at the same time. I don't want her to have anesthesia twice."

I schedule Tara's surgery for the following Thursday and her pre-op blood work for the coming Monday. So much for the hiatus of no vet bills, procedures, and anxiety. I call Laura to make an appointment to come talk to the dogs and explain to Tara what is happening. I call Amanda to schedule baths for all three.

In the past two weeks Kundun's arthritis has taken a nasty turn. He can barely move, has trouble getting in and out of his crate where the bio-pad is, and it is painful to watch him lie down with small halted movements toward the floor then a final flop.

Laura arrives to talk to Tara about her upcoming surgery, "You have a lump on your back and it needs to be removed."

"I got hit by an acorn."

"Rasa, you can tell Tara about what to expect."

"They put a tube down your throat and in your nose."

"How do you know that?"

"I was in a pen next to where they do it."

I realize that this had to be where she had her dental surgery. "No wonder she started trying to chew on the chain link while in there!" SHE HAD TO WATCH!

"You throw up. They tell you it's okay. You have a big headache the next day."

Kundun offers, "Bumps grow so fast. You go to the vet, get it removed. It comes back and you have to go back to the vet."

"I'm sure he remembers when Rasa went back for surgery after two weeks. They all seem sad, why?"

"I don't want anyone to hurt. I think of Laura and she is sad," Kundun answers.

Laura's wolf-dog, Maia, died recently. My neighbor just died of cancer, and my mother died of cancer at the same age—fifty-seven. I always knew that was young, but now that I am older than that, I really understand how young it is.

Kundun says, "I am worried about my mom dying. I see her mom sitting at the table with her. She says, 'Read this article, that book'. Sometimes she sits behind Mom and says, 'That's a clever way to say that!' I wish Mom could see her."

Tara adds, "I could see angels with her when I saw the neighbor, so I knew she was going to die. There were angels all around the house in Pecos, and when I was kicked an angel stopped his foot and knocked him down."

"Why didn't you tell me that before?" Laura asks.

"I forgot about it until we were talking about angels. I see an angel standing behind you now."

Rasa says, "My mom's mother is here a lot lately."

"How often?" Laura asks.

"More than we take a walk."

"Will an angel come with me to surgery?"

"Yes, definitely!" I exclaim.

"What else you guys?"

"Kundun got to see the new young coyotes. I think they are Chatty's."

"I am going to be friends with them."

"Tara, what do you think about being friends?"

"I think they have germs and should stay away."

Rasa adds, "I'm not going to be friends—I'm going to chase them away."

Tara moves over to Laura, sits next to her leg, and looks up at her, "I'm not scared of you anymore. I'm going to be your friend."

"Any questions for Mom?"

Kundun asks, "How does Genji get thrush and what does he need to treat it?"

Tano was at the stable to shoe Genji an hour before our session with Laura. Kundun was not with me when I drove out to pay Tano. I looked at Genji's hooves without shoes, and we discussed the thrush problem, which has been ongoing for two years. Laura and I explain to Kundun that Genji gets thrush from standing in wet ground from his water tank being emptied in the corral, and from rain, and it is treated with a special product that is applied to his hooves.

Tara pipes up, "The full moon makes people angry—the gardner got angry at the hose."

Tara wasn't home on the day the landscape maintenance man was here. She, Rasa, and Kundun were having baths. This is probably the most amazing thing I've encountered with the dogs and Genji. They know what is happening when they aren't physically present. They communicate with each other, me, and scope the territory with their minds. It's a phenomenal concept to comprehend.

"There are holes in the universe," states Rasa.

"She sounds like Stephen Hawking." I'm looking at her in surprise.

"What about questions?"

"I can answer all of the questions myself. Black holes are like crinkled paper. You want to go where it's like a light zipper."

I look at her, "How do you know these things?"

"With no walks, I just think all of the time."

"I slack off on walks and you're becoming a quantum physicist?!"

"We all have teachers who come to us when we're sleeping and teach us things."

"Is that the same as dreaming?"

"It's like a guided dream."

I ride Genji on Sunday. After a tender-footed first one hundred feet from the barn, I turn him around and head for the large covered arena. As it has in the past, the soft sandy arena surface masks his problem for a while. Then there it is, the unmistakable right front leg going out of gait, his slowing down, and back to the barn we go.

When I arrive for the dog bath appointment, I ask Amanda if she knows of a vet who is a chiropractor. Amanda's grooming facility is in the back of The American Hay Company in Oak View. "Funny you should ask, a new veterinarian just posted a flyer on the bulletin board right there, and he does chiropractic work."

I read the flyer and take the phone number. He not only works on horses, he does dog chiropractic work as well. I make an appointment with Dr. Monroe *Vet. Chiro.* to meet at the stable Friday to treat both Genji and Kundun.

Thursday morning is Tara's surgery day. She is frisky and adorable about breakfast. However, Tara cannot eat or even drink water this morning. I have a routine to deal with feeding two dogs and not the one going to surgery. I put Tara in the SUV and open the rear windows. It is cool, so she will be fine until we leave. I go back inside to feed Rasa and Kundun, clean up, and leave at seven.

"You are going to be fine Tara. I know you don't like Dr. Nicci, but she is an excellent surgeon and you'll be okay. There will be an angel with you all day, Tara, maybe two."

We arrive at Buena a few minutes early. I sign the paperwork and watch Tara reluctantly follow the vet tech. "I love you, Tara." I drive home worried about everything: anesthesia at her age, whether the lump is cancer, if it's cancer that they get it all.

Later in the morning the call comes from Buena, "Tara is fine. She is coming out of anesthesia. You can pick her up at five."

I am relieved. I arrive at five. The vet tech hands me a white paper bag with her antibiotics in it. The bags always have the dog's name and a heart drawn in color marker pen, which is very sweet. Tara comes out with the soft collar I provided. She walks to the car, but can't get in. I lift all sixty-five pounds of her up and into the back door. She goes limp and collapses right where I have lifted and pushed her as far as I can. At home she won't move to get out of the car. She is lying on her stomach on a large towel, so I grab both sides of the towel and pull her out back end first. She won't walk. I struggle with the towel lifting and dragging her. I can feel my lower back being destroyed. Once in the house door, I straddle her and continue to drag and pull. Throw rugs catch under her back feet and come with us until I feel like I'm dragging one hundred pounds. I get Tara to her bed and somehow get her into it. I am in pain and it's time to feed everyone dinner. Tara refuses food.

In the morning I find Tara lying on the throw rug next to her bed. She has peed right there. She still won't move. I remove the post-surgical collar, and she immediately stands up and walks. Her protest was extremely effective.

I meet Dr. Monroe at the stable. I decide to have him give Kundun a treatment first. In the past two weeks Kundun's mobility has become extremely compromised. He seems to be a little better after Steve's adjustment of his atlas vertebra, and then a week later he got worse. His butt is curling under. His back legs are becoming more and more bent. His front right foot is turning sideways. He can barely stand on three legs to pee. His head has no upward movement, so he can no longer howl with the coyotes, and he has an old man shuffle to his gait. Worse of all, there is no big grin on his face anymore. Suddenly he stopped playing with Rasa in the kitchen after dinner last week. He isn't at the bottom of the stairs all excited waiting for me in the morning.

Dr. Monroe adjusts his back and his treatment seems fairly stress-free until he does an adjustment behind his shoulders that makes Kundun scream in pain, snap his jaws like a shark and turn back to bite the vet, who jumps away. As Kundun's head swings back around toward me, a tooth grazes my wrist as I jump back. Of course, all of the ranch dogs swarm over Kundun as if in for the kill. I am not expecting anything this radical in a treatment and am shocked. I am so stunned by what has happened I freeze. I don't yell at this crazy vet. He says nothing as if this is normal.

Dr. Monroe works on Genji, and his treatment seems to go well. Kundun stands on the grass in front of the stall looking at me very apprehensively. When we leave, he can barely get in the car. I have to help him. When we get home it takes a lot of coaxing to get him out. He is trembling and shaking. I am terrified.

After the weekend I know that Kundun's treatment was far too intense. He quits eating in the mornings, has loose stools, and looks at me continuously with deep, dark brown eyes. He won't even eat treats now. After much coaxing with petting and talking I get him to take Tara's pain pills with his thyroid medication as well as something for digestion.

I call Dr. Monroe and he asks, "How is Kundun doing?"

"He is much worse. You hurt him horribly"

"The life expectancy for this breed is nine to eleven years, and Kundun is eleven now. The loose stools should only have been during the first twenty-four hours. You need to take him to your regular vet."

I hang up absolutely furious. I make an appointment for Kundun at Buena. I call Laura to come talk to Kundun.

The biopsy report comes back and Tara's lump is a tumor—a low grade soft tissue spindle cell neuro-fibro sarcoma. It was completely *incised—no cancer is left at the site. I make an appointment with Dr. Alice for a consultation.

Then I have a dream. Wuli is with one of my dogs and I accidently lock them in a dark, old garage. I don't have a key, and I can't get them out. I look for a key in a stranger's home nearby and I am discovered frantically rummaging through drawers looking for a key. Oh my God, I dreamed about Wuli! Which dog was with her? I think about the dream all day and I cannot see the other dog. It looked shadowy and ghostly, and was trapped in that dark, dingy place. I feel scared and helpless as a wave of panic washes over me.

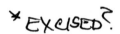 * EXCISED?.

30

ecause Kundun can no longer duck into the large crate, I have removed it from the kitchen into the garage. The bio-pad which was in the crate is still on the bed that was in the crate, but they are on the floor next to the island counter and cupboard not far from my chair at the end of the table. The new arrangement of dog beds has created a new dynamic. Tara has voluntarily begun to lie on the bio-pad. Because of her terror of a crate after her experience on the ranch, she would never go into the crate here in the kitchen. Because there are now three choices for beds, not four, the musical beds dance doesn't work. The dog bed from my office is now in the corner where the crate used to be and it is huge, so Rasa will actually get on this bed with Kundun. Rasa has absolutely never done this in her entire life. She would provoke Kundun into moving so that she could take over whatever bed she wanted if he was on it.

We have our appointment with Cynthia. After calling her to explain that Kundun will not be able to go up and down the stairs to her second story office, she moves her office into the living room for us. I help Kundun in and out of the car. He makes it up the four steps to her door with enthusiastic coaching. The living room is furnished with Victorian furniture and an over-sized dark leather chair with a matching ottoman. Cynthia conducts our session from here.

"Kundun is detoxing prevacox. He is allergic to all COX-2 inhibitors. The loose stools and not eating indicate that his liver is working to cleanse his body." Cynthia makes us all feel comfortable in her cozy home at the end of what has been a night and day of steady rain with a crisp, cool autumn feel to the air. Misty clouds cling to the mountain sides and tops surrounding the valley.

In the morning when I walk into the kitchen I notice that the throw rug in front of the stove is turned up on one end. "That's strange," I think. I turn the corner around the island and there is Kundun spread-eagled on the floor unable to move. I put Rasa outside and return to Kundun. I try to help him onto his feet by putting my arms around his mid-section and lifting up. His back legs don't work. I retrieve a bath size towel from the laundry room, fold it into thirds and get it under him like a sling. I lift him up off his back legs while he is attempting to use his front legs. I realize that I have no idea where I'm trying to move him. I put him down a few feet from where he was and place a worn thin fleece bed on the floor near the huge bed and the door. He has slept on this leopard-patterned fleece pad on top of other beds and pads most of his life. I struggle and get most of his body on it.

After feeding Rasa and Tara and making my tea, I sit in my kitchen chair and burst into tears. I call Laura and leave a message, "Tomorrow won't be soon enough for our session. Can you please come as soon as possible?"

Kundun's entire body is shaking. He hasn't eaten for thirty-six hours. He won't drink, not even lick water off my fingers. I place a folded up hand towel under his chin because he seems so uncomfortable trying to put his head down. By the time I shower, dress, eat a bowl of granola, and wash dishes, it is time for Laura to arrive.

Rasa and Tara greet Laura at the door. "Hi, how are you guys?" Laura laughs, "Tara says it's a good thing we told her what to expect—she really felt sick after surgery."

Laura kneels next to Kundun and has a silent conversation with him. "He is in horrible, unbelievable pain."

"My back and neck are in pain. I don't want to die like this. I want to die happy."

Rasa emphatically states, "When it's this painful—I say get a doctor!"

Tara is lying in her bed watching Kundun, "This is so scary—get him to the hospital!"

Kundun continues, "I'm sick to my stomach and feel nausea. I don't want to go to Heaven yet. If I die, tell my mom I love her."

"Kundun, I love you too."

"When you're sick you have to keep saying, 'Get better.'" Rasa instructs.

"I can't handle this." Tara's eyes are big and frightened looking. I've never seen her look like this.

Laura and I discuss what to do.

"I think Kundun needs to go to the nearest vet as soon as possible."

"I'll only take him to Buena, it's a twenty minute drive. Will you help me get him in my car?"

We walk out to my car and determine how we will do it. We carry the car dog bed into the kitchen. Laura explains to Kundun what we are doing. The towel I used earlier in the morning is still under him. We use that to lift him onto the car bed. We each grab an end. I am shocked at how light he seems. In January he weighed ninety pounds. I put him on a diet and he lost eight pounds in three months. When he became ill in July he weighed seventy-five pounds. Now I guess that he doesn't weigh over sixty pounds. We get him in the car with much lifting, pulling and pushing. Laura and I hug and say goodbye.

I drive west on Creek Road, turn left on Highway 33 to the 101, then south to the Telephone Street exit and Buena Animal Hospital on Main Street. I park in front of the door, open the back, and go in. I had called before leaving, so we are expected. A vet tech comes to the car and gets information about everything in his life for the past five days. He disappears into the clinic. I sit on the tailgate and rub Kundun's ears, stroke his head and neck, and tell him I love him. Two vet techs return with a stretcher, pull him onto it, strap him in, and carry him inside as I watch helplessly.

When I get home, I already have a message from Dr. Nicci. "Hi, this is Dr. Nicci. Kundun has encephalitis with a high fever. He has neurological deficits in all four limbs, neck pain and back pain. Call me as soon as you get this message."

Like a zombie, I dial the number, "Hello, this is Louise, Dr. Nicci said to call immediately."

"I'm going to start emergency therapy immediately. I will slam him with steroids and antibiotics. Encephalitis is an inflammation of the spinal cord and brain. This is a rare disease. It's unusual that he has it. His temperature is 104.4. Normal is 102.5. There are several things that can cause this. It can be bacterial or immune mediated. In Kundun's case, I believe it is immune mediated because of what happened to him before. The big problem is that to treat the encephalitis we have to use prednisone, and when we used prednisone to treat his autoimmune problem with his gums, that is what caused his gastro-intestinal issues in July. And, he will still have his arthritis."

"Kundun said that he doesn't want to die like this. He wants to die happy. I want you to try to make him happy."

"Then this is what I think you should do. I will get him walking hopefully. I will try to eliminate his pain. You can take him home and have a couple of weeks with him, then he needs to be euthanized." By now Dr. Nicci is crying.

I am crying, "Okay, I need to think about this. I'll talk to you tomorrow. Thank you. Bye"

I drive to Suzanne's for lunch. I cry the entire way. I eat lunch here every day except Tuesday when they are closed. Everyone who works the lunch shift is friend, family. I am fed well, and looked after with great detail—water with no ice, a slice of lemon and a slice of lime; one slice of bread, not two with olive oil, not butter. When I tell Jason about Kundun he buys me a Margarita. I feel better while I'm there, but I cry all the way home.

The house is a little too quiet without Mr. K. He has a huge presence without making a sound. Rasa and Tara seem at odds without the whole family together. I'm having a premonition of life without him after almost eleven years.

Dr. Nicci calls at six P.M. I have his pain cut in half, now we're trying to get him to eat something. Do you want to come see him tomorrow?"

"Yes, in the morning."

"I'll be in surgery all morning, but hopefully you'll be here when I have a moment to see you."

I spend half the night awake with thoughts of Kundun, of how eleven years flashed by, of how robust and strong he was, and how fragile and weak he is now. Rasa and Tara sleep deeply, while crushing thoughts of losing each of my special pals take over my mind. I can't bear wondering how empty and silent that will be.

31

I arrive at Buena later than I had said I'd be there on Friday morning. I have Rasa and Tara in the car with me, because after I visit Kundun I plan to take them for a walk.

"We have a room all ready for you. Come this way."

I don't know what I was expecting. I thought I would go into the back to the kennel area like I had when Kundun was here in July. I walk into the room. A fleece blanket is on top of a pad on the floor. Then two vet techs bring in Kundun. One rolls the IV stand with the tube connected to his front leg and one holds the sling around his abdomen to keep his hindquarters up while Kundun haltingly walks with his front legs. They arrange him on the bed and leave. I crouch down by his head and stroke him. He is still shaking, but not quite as bad as yesterday. He is extremely thin and I finally realize that this is it. He will not walk again. He is not coming home again. Dr. Nicci comes in to the room in her surgical gown.

"I had hoped we could get him walking again and he could go home for a couple of weeks. I recommend that you have him euthanized."

I nod my head, "I decided that as soon as I saw him."

She holds out a box of Kleenex and I take several. We discuss how she does an euthanasia. "I want it done tomorrow, and I want him cremated." Dr. Nicci leaves the room to give her staff instructions and to return to surgery. When the staff hears the news, different vet techs and office personnel come in to hug me. Everyone here loves Kundun.

I pet and stroke Kundun's head and rub his great big soft ears, "It's time to go to Heaven, Kundun. No one wants to die. I don't want to lose you, but you're never going to get better, Kundun. There's a whole pack of spirit dogs waiting for you, and you won't be in pain any more. I know you want to die happy. We all want to die happy, but this is it, we don't always have a choice. I'm sorry Kundun. I'm so sorry." I open the door and ask a vet tech to watch him, "I'm going to bring Rasa and Tara in to visit him. They're in the car. I'll be right back."

We go into the room. Rasa immediately sniffs Kundun's head and neck. Tara's eyes are big and she touches his face with her nose. Rasa eats the treat that Dr. Nicci left for Kundun that he wouldn't eat. I laugh. Rasa never misses any food laying around. After some time together, Kundun is moved out of the room. Rasa, Tara and I get in the car and leave.

I park on the street next to the state park near the beach that Kundun calls the big grass. "Okay girls, this walk is for Kundun. I know he knows we're here." I remember the last time I brought him here in August. I walked him all the way across the park. It was too much for him, and on the way back he walked slower and slower and began to pant. I felt concerned about making it back to the car.

I forget the plastic bags for the poop, and sure enough Tara stops to poop. I see a stray plastic bag under a picnic table and retrieve it. It's wet and muddy from the rain, but I take it back to dispose of the poop. I don't realize it but the bag has a hole in it and I stick my finger through the hole and into the poop while I am scooping it up. I walk to the nearest trash can and throw in the bag. I look at my hand, squat down, dig my fingers through the dirt, wipe them on the grass and continue on our walk while trying to hold the leashes with one hand. I spot another bag and grab it for Rasa. Then I see a faucet and try to rinse off my hand. I accomplish all of this without uttering one sound. Two years ago I would have let out a stream of four letter words, gotten completely pissed, and scared my dogs. Today I just laugh and deal with it. I reflect on my transformation.

After we return home, I call Laura to tell her about Kundun and my decision to euthanize him in the morning. She promises to communicate with him later tonight and call me in the morning.

I am just stepping into the shower when the phone rings. I get Laura's message, "Hi Louise this is Laura. I spoke to Kundun and he said he's ready. He's been seeing angels and spirits around him and feels already partially in Heaven. He's ready, wants me to tell you he's ready, that he loves you, and thank you for everything. He wants you to sit with him before the euthanasia. I'm trying to cancel an appointment to go see him this morning."

I play her message several times. "Thank you for everything." "No, Kundun, thank *you* for everything!" Rasa and Tara watch as tears cascade from my eyes. The house is too quiet without Kundun. His tail was always thumping against something—his bed, his crate, the kitchen cabinets, doors, walls. He had such a huge presence, and now the space seems too big for just the three of us. He held us all together and I didn't even realize it.

32

I drive to Ventura with Rasa and Tara. It's a beautiful day. The sky is blue, the Channel Islands are visible, and the ocean is deep azure and calm. It is seventy-two degrees, which is warm for Ventura. We arrive at Buena. A vet tech comes to my car, which I park under the overhang in front of the entrance. I give her Kundun's worn out leopard patterned bed that he has had on top of various pads and beds most of his life. "I want Kundun on this pad." I hand her a galvanized metal vase with flowers in it.

"Laura was able to come see Kundun this morning."

"Oh, wonderful," I respond.

We go into the room. Tara begins to shake out of fear. Kundun's pile of blankets with his leopard pad on top are arranged on the floor. I make an impromptu altar on the operating table with a candle, the flowers, and a bundle of white sage. I realize that I overlooked bringing a small Buddha. I have the CD we've listened to every morning for years. A small CD player is waiting in the room for it, and soon the haunting, melancholy music surrounds us. The door opens and a vet tech carries Kundun to the leopard bed, gets him settled then leaves.

As soon as I see him I say, "Oh hello Kundun." He looks fragile, diminished, a shadow of himself. With a stab of nausea at the pit of my stomach, I now see the other dog in my dream. I sit down beside him with my legs out in front of me. I bend over and kiss him on his head. I pet him, hug him, cry, talk to him. Rasa doesn't like Kundun getting all of this attention. She sticks her face in mine and I hug her too. Rasa and Tara both lie down. I don't want to light the sage in the clinic, so I smudge Kundun without smoke. Rasa butts in—she wants to be smudged also. I smudge all of us. Kundun seems to relax. He stops shaking. He lays his head down.

Dr. Nicci comes into the room. "We're ready now," I tell her. She leaves and returns with the hypodermic needles. Kundun has his IV cuff on his leg and she injects the first drug which is like an anesthesia. He slowly slumps down. I pull his head onto my thigh, bend over his head with my arms around him and sob uncontrollably. I realize that Rasa is standing right next to me on my left side. I put my arm around her and pull her close to my side. Kundun is deep asleep and snoring. Dr. Nicci picks up the second needle, and I exclaim, "Oh no!"

"We'll wait," she says.

I breathe, "Okay, now."

She listens with her stethoscope, and looks at me. "His heart has stopped."

I continue to stroke his head, but he is gone, so I gently place his head on the pad between his front legs, feel his ears for the last time, and get up. I gather all of the stuff I brought, take Rasa's and Tara's leashes and start toward the door. I stop, turn, and look back. His ears are standing up, his eyes are open, and he looks so peaceful lying on his leopard pad like he's ready to jump up and come with us. After what he has been through this past week, it's a memorable last image of him. I have requested a private cremation for him and maybe one day will make a pilgrimage to the big land with his ashes.

Back at home it is empty and quiet without him. A wave of loneliness washes over me. I think to myself that if I can just try to be like Kundun was with his selfless big heart, unconditional love, happy smile, endless enthusiasm, concern for the rest of us, never giving up, living in the moment—I'll be a very good person.

After dark when I have Rasa and Tara out for their last potty break at the edge of the huge oaks, a lone coyote begins to howl. He sounds like he is just on the other side of the fence across the grove. Maybe it is Chatty saying goodbye to Kundun, because I haven't heard coyotes for a while, and that is where they met a short two years ago.

Kundun runs up to me. I reach out to touch him. I run my hands down his back. I pet him and stroke his body. My hands begin to sink into his form. His body fades into invisibility until my hands and arms are merely flailing in air. I wake and grasp at the fragments. Oh, Kundun.

33

aura arrives six days after Kundun's death and hands me a card. While we sit at the kitchen table, Laura checks in with Rasa and Tara. I read her card,

"Dear Louise,

My animal family and I are sending you lots of love and light. We know how empty the house must feel. Please find comfort that Kundun is soaring in the dimensions above. He is watching over all of you, protecting you and creating miracles—another angel on your side. You will meet each other again whether both in body or both in spirit. In the meanwhile you are connected by a golden ribbon that cannot be broken.

Much love, Laura"

Tara speaks up first, "I see Kundun sometimes and he has a furry dog with him."

I ask, "What color is it?"

"Light brown," Laura says.

"Maybe that is Jasmine, my red Chow."

Tara continues, "Kundun told me when I leave my skin I'll leave behind my problems. I saw his spirit turn into a flickering light."

"When he died?" I ask, already knowing the answer.

Laura nods yes.

"I can't see Kundun as a body, but he is there as a friend," Tara finishes.

"How are you doing, Tara?" I ask.

"I'm doing fine. I want slurpier food. I want a fence in front, so I can go out there. I think you should put water somewhere else on the property because rodents are drinking out of the fountain at night. You should read to me what you've written so I can tell you if it sounds good."

Rasa, who has been quiet so far now speaks out, "I also saw a flickering light when Kundun died. Kundun tells me to smile and be happy, take care of Mom. The hardest part is when Mom is gone from home and I feel lonely. I miss

DEATH AS RELEASE
FROM SUFFERING.

his thumping, thumping tail. It used to annoy me, but now I miss the sound. When I see Kundun, I want to see him in body, but he says he doesn't need a body. Why did he leave us?"

"He told me he'd see me in spirit before body," Tara adds.

"I'm upset that Kundun was in the hospital. I didn't like him being there. I thought he should have been here with us. Can I have more gravy in my food too?"

"Okay, let's talk to Kundun!" Laura closes her eyes and bows her head slightly. Her eyelids move.

"I didn't really want to die, so I was fighting it. My passing was very peaceful. I saw Mom's mother right away. She took me to a country with rolling green hills, and fed me a beef stew. I want to be your teacher and teach you how to heal with your hands. When you meditate look at the light coming from the center of your palms."

"Oh, your mother is here," Laura exclaims.

Ruth interrupts with, "Cassidy will get pregnant in four months and eight days. An older handsome doctor will help her."

"Don't pay any attention to the timeframe—it doesn't mean anything," Laura adds.

Kundun continues, "It was like an echoing chamber at the vet. I heard murmuring voices on the land at home, but I didn't know it then. There is a lot of restless movement there.

"I miss you, Kundun. I didn't think it was time for you to die yet either. I love you and I miss your thumping tail."

"I'll start thumping my tail again when I get stronger from the energy around me. You need to walk more."

"Dr. Nicci says to say, 'Hello.'"

"She has very gentle hands and an angel that is with her to help her do this."

"Don't worry, the things that scare you—Kundun is watching us," Tara tells me.

I do feel vulnerable, and it worries me that Kundun isn't here to guard the downstairs now.

Kundun has one last thing to tell me, "I can hear you when you talk to me."

34

oday is Tara's consultation appointment with Dr. Alice Villalobos for her cancer and potential treatment. I take Rasa also for moral support for Tara, to say hello to Dr. Alice and her staff, and because I don't want to leave her home alone. Tara is weighed—fifty-eight pounds and we are ushered into a room. I am handed a sheet of paper titled, "Soft Tissue Sarcomas (STS)." I read it and my heart skips a few beats, "Soft tissue sarcomas may grow anywhere, but are seen most commonly in the skin and subcutaneous tissues...STS's often kill senior and geriatric dogs because they are initially underestimated."

Dr. Alice enters the room with a woman who is filming a documentary. Rasa, Tara and I are introduced to Marilyn Braverman. Dr. Alice explains to her that it is not uncommon for two dogs in the same family to develop cancer. Dr. Alice has her clients answer two questions on a form before she initiates a regimen for the dog. The first question is, "What do you know about your dog's cancer?" The second question is what do you want to accomplish for your dog?" She has me go over my experience with Tara's cancer for the film. I show her where I found the button-sized hard bump and how I felt it every night before going to bed. I explain how it suddenly became large and irregular shaped, and alarmed I immediately took her to the vet.

The answer to the second question is read aloud by Dr. Alice. "Because of Tara's age and her fragile emotional state, I don't want to put her on chemo. I am here to discuss supplements and other options." Dr. Alice sits next to me on a bench, and Rasa places her head in her lap. She looks up at Dr. Alice with clear blue eyes, tail wagging. Her entire body shaking, Tara leans against my legs.

"Radiation is very good for this kind of cancer, but it is expensive and her tumor is right above her kidneys and liver. The radiation can damage them. Another option is what we call carboplatin. We draw blood, spin it to eliminate the blood cells, then mix that serum with one-tenth of the strength of what is used for intravenous chemo-therapy. This mixture is then injected all around the incision area. The needle can go into the tissue deeper that the scalpel did for the surgery. We will do this in four sessions."

"I am interested in this option."

Tara is ushered out of the room for her first treatment. Dr. Alice goes over the supplement regimen. She increases all that I am giving her presently and adds two more. I am relieved that there is a way to give Tara a treatment without months of chemo, steroids, intestinal upset, aggressive behavior, and everything else that I went through with Rasa. I only need to drive to Woodland Hills an hour away on Highway 101 four times. We figure out a schedule of three treatments before Thanksgiving and one in December.

It is a windy day. The Santa Ana wind is blowing off the Mojave Desert, down the mountains, and through the Sespe River Valley to the ocean. These are the warm dry winds that create wildfire situations in California. I love the story about how the Santa Ana winds acquired their name. When California was still part of Mexico, the Mexican general, Santa Ana, moved his army which included the military, their families, the livestock for food, wagons and ammunition. This huge entity stirred up dust clouds that could be seen for miles and miles. So, now we have the well named Santa Ana winds, a whisper of history in the present.

I have one stop on the way home. Kundun's ashes are ready to pick up at Buena. When I walk in the door, one of the vet techs calls, "Ms. Heydt".

I turn toward her, "Yes?"

"I watched a special on TV about the Dalai Lama—Kundun. Kundun, your dog. I always thought Kundun was such a strong name, and it's the Dalai Lama's name! I had no idea. It's funny how you learn things."

I place the bag with Kundun's ashes on the seat next to me for the drive home. Once there, I get Rasa and Tara settled then pull all of the tissue out of the bag. On top of the box of ashes is something round and heavy. What is this, I wonder? I open it, and there is Kundun's paw print in plaster with his name and a little shiny star. I take the rectangular cedar box out of the bag and hold it in my lap. His name is on the top in brass, and on the front is a little brass lock with two tiny keys. I burst into tears at the sight of the keys.

I place his paw print in the center of the circle of his buckled collar on my altar in my meditation room. I bought him this collar in Santa Fe many years ago. It is beaded by African Masais in desert-like tones of bronze, gold, and white, much like the colors of his brindle coat. I place his box of ashes in the kitchen in the niche in the rock wall of the fireplace where I have placed all of the crystals and a dancing bronze Ganesha that I acquired in Kuala Lompur. All of the sympathy cards that I received on his behalf are placed in there as well. Everyone loved Kundun.

35

Not here in L.A.

The letter that arrives with Kundun's ashes includes information about their grief support program, which is complimentary for cremation clients. After struggling with my guilt, inability to sleep, or eat, and my despair over Kundun's death for a month, I call to make an appointment.

Dr. Kathleen Ayl meets with me in a small, cozy, windowless room at the VSMG emergency clinic in Ventura. She is a specialist in pet loss support, and has been for ten years. She has me fill out some information on a form. Dr. Ayl is slender and attractive with sparkling eyes and a clear voice. At first we talk in generalities about losing a pet and the grief. She explains some of her background such as living in India for three years and working with Mother Teresa.

"The main reason that I am here today is to talk about a chiropractic treatment that I had a vet do on Kundun. He hurt my dog horribly. I took Kundun to the stable because I was also having this vet do a treatment on my horse. I decided to have him work on Kundun first. We were on the lawn in front of Genji's barn. The treatment seemed fairly straight forward and gentle— then the vet did something right behind Kundun's shoulder blades. Kundun snapped his jaws together twice, screamed in pain and lunged back toward the vet with his mouth wide open and teeth bared. Then he turned toward me jaws snapping, huge white teeth grazing my arm. I said, "not me," and jumped back. As soon as this all happened four ranch dogs jumped him. I was so worried that they would attack and injure him, my mind froze. I did not yell, "What the hell are you doing?" In a trance, I let him continue working on Kundun's front leg.

By now Kathleen's face is reflecting the horror of this nightmare story. "I want to know his name so I can make sure no clients of ours take their dogs to him."

"I feel so guilty about this, because Kundun could get in the car to go to the stable, but I had to help him get in to leave. The following morning he couldn't get down the hill back to the kitchen door. I saw this and went outside in my bathrobe to talk him down. By Monday he was having serious problems walking, trying to stand on three legs to pee, and squatting to poop. He could no longer duck down the two inches to get in and out of his crate. My housekeeper and I moved it out of the kitchen and into the garage. I called Dr. Monroe to tell him Kundun was worse. He responded, 'This is his breed's life expectancy.' I asked, what about the pain? He said, 'I think I released something.' I hung up completely furious and astonished. So, I lie in bed every night saying, I'm sorry Kundun. I'm sorry. I'm sorry Kundun, I'm sorry. I can't sleep. I keep visualizing that entire violent scene and it's my fault. I am filled with guilt. No one ever hurt him in his entire lucky life with me until this."

Kathleen responds, "You have post-traumatic stress disorder. Change your mantra from 'I'm sorry' to 'I tried to do the right thing, I tried to help.'"

I thank Kathleen for talking to me and drive home. I think of how things have changed so much. I can seek grief counseling for losing my beloved dog. Indeed, Dr. Ayl has a career based on pet loss grief.

Kundun instructs me, "Tell me, 'I love you, not I'm sorry.'"

As I do that the sorry fades and the love radiates.

This is good

for me, + Chachi.

No more Hóoponopono!

36

oday it is five weeks since Kundun left us. Laura and I meet at the stable. When she arrives I have Genji in his halter and he is eagerly eating new shoots of green grass that have appeared after a November rain.

"Genji has an exciting story to tell—he escaped from his stall!"

"How did you do that?"

"I opened the gate."

"Genji, I think that is so funny. It must not have been hooked. I always double-check it before I leave, and I was here three days ago."

"What time did you get out? Was it dark?" Laura asks.

"It was night."

"What did you do? Where did you go?"

"I ate grass. I walked down the aisle of the big barn. I visited other horses. I invited them to come out and join me. One horse kicked the fence, but couldn't get out."

"Thank goodness nothing happened to you!"

"I tried to go back in my stall, but the gate was closed." Genji continues to graze while we are having our conversation.

"Genji became ill. He developed colic a week ago. He was being shod and kept acting strangely. Tano and I thought the flies were bothering him, so we kept spraying him with fly repellant. He repeatedly rested his chin on Tano's back, and having one foot up on the stand to work on his hoof seemed to bother him. After Tano was finished I walked him back to his stall. I put the fly spray in the tack room. When I returned two minutes later he was lying down and the apples that I had left as a treat in his feeder were uneaten. I brought Tano to his stall and we observed him together. After he stood up he kept trying to hit at his belly with a back foot. We concluded it was colic and I called a vet."

"Oh, Genji, how are you feeling now?"

"It was hot and then it was cold and it made me sick."

"Horses don't always drink enough water when the temperature does this. Their food gets compacted in the intestines which causes a blockage."

"I have a good mom who takes good care of me. There are horses here that don't have good moms. Spirits come at night to be with these horses."

"What do these spirits look like?"

"They look like veterinarians your age. I saw them while I was out."

"Did you know about them before?"

"No, I am usually asleep. They tell these horses that they will have good moms in their next life."

"Not until then?"

"No, they have to live this life with the moms they have."

"Did these spirits know each other while they were living?"

"The spirits didn't know each other until they met in Heaven. They formed a group to do this work."

"Wow" is my response to this exchange between Laura and Genji.

"Genji, how are you doing with your supplements?" I ask.

"I want more."

"Do you mean different supplements or more of what you have?" Laura questions.

"More of what I have."

Laura explains, "When the weather gets colder, many horses ask for more supplements. How is his hoof? I see a big chip right there."

"I'm going to change his hoof supplement, he's been having this problem lately."

"How are your feet, Genji?"

"My feet feel fine it's my shoulder that bothers me."

"That's why we're not riding. Genji is resting his shoulder and I am resting my back."

"Do you have a bad back?"

"I had a fall off my Tennessee Walking Horse mare, Sunny, when I was in my mid-twenties. Two vertebrae cracked and the disc between them ruptured. Several years later I had major back surgery to repair the ruptured disc. The doctors told me that I'd never ski, or ride a horse, or do anything athletic again. As you can see I proved them wrong."

"I want you to ride me bareback in the arena!"

"How about the English saddle?"

"A bareback pad."

"I've never ridden bareback since my accident over forty years ago."

"I want you to read me a book. I'm bored."

"Okay, Genji, I promise I will get a chair, put it in your stall, and read to you about Sea Bisquit's races."

"Are you going to read it aloud or in your head?" Laura asks me.

"I had planned to read it aloud."

Laura confers with Genji about the aloud so the other horses hear it.

"Read it aloud, we are all bored, and then we can talk about it later."

I decide that sounds like fun and I don't really care if everyone out here thinks I'm crazy. "I'll read to you next week."

"Do you want to talk to Kundun?"

"Oh yes!"

"I'm helping Ganesha."

I don't grasp this at first. His comment goes right over my head.

"Don't you have a Ganesha in your meditation room?" Laura asks.

"Yes, I do. And I placed Kundun's ashes in that niche in the kitchen with all of the crystals and a dancing Ganesha. As you probably know, Ganesha is the remover of obstacles."

"I am behind the obstacles."

"That takes a fairly highly evolved being to be Ganesha's helper, don't you think?"

The impact of this finally sinks in, "You know I always thought Kundun was special, but this is mind-blowing."

"I look like Ganesha."

Laura and I laugh. "He has big ears."

"Genji, how do you feel about Kundun's passing?"

"I miss seeing him in his body form."

"What does he look like to you now?"

"He looks like a shooting star."

"Kundun, there is a buyer for the big land."

"I showed her a couple of our secret trails and a secret place."

"Oh, you already know!"

"Kundun says to take Rasa and Tara to a big park," Genji adds. "Kundun made Mom laugh and be happy."

"I miss my clown. I'm trying to laugh and be happy."

Kundun responds, "Instead of saying, 'I'm sorry' say I love you!"

"I do say I love you. I'll say it more."

"I don't like getting older," Genji states.

"Neither do I," I agree.

Genji asks, "When will I die?"

"We don't know that," Laura answers.

"Oh, does Genji know Natasha is leaving? She is getting married."

I am beginning to understand now that maybe always, but for certain sometimes, a very particular dog will come into our lives, and perhaps it is a Bodhisattva who has chosen to reincarnate in any form to enlighten a soul living in a body. I believe Kundun is such a Bodhisattva. He was pure love in his dog-body-form-life. You simply could not know him without feeling happy and laughing. His thumping tail was the music of his life in our home. If I didn't pet him before he went out in the morning, before placing his food dish in front of him—then his day wasn't working and he wouldn't eat. He would get in his crate and look sad. So, if you don't think that kiss, that hug, that pat is important—I have news. If you don't think a happy voice is setting the frequency for the day—think again. If you are out of tune with yourself, believe me—a dog like Kundun with one look can send you scrambling for balance and equanimity.

I am grateful for this lesson.

How does it feel to find out that your dog in the afterlife is Ganesha's assistant? I am humbled. I can never rub Ganesha's trunk again without acknowledging that Kundun is behind the obstacles. There are hundreds of millions of humans praying to Ganesha to remove obstacles to accomplish this or that. And he lived with me for eleven years! Why me? I cannot answer these questions. I can only feel blessed, be a better, more evolved person from my experience, and try to understand that God touched my life in a very special way to guide me on the way to enlightenment.

37

In the time since Kundun's passing things shift almost imperceptibly. Tara spends more time outside, and becomes her former silly self in the house being playful and rolling on her back to have her chest and tummy rubbed. She seems more confident. Rasa joins Tara outside now that the days are cooler. The house is quieter without Kundun beginning to get excited the second he heard Rasa's front feet hit the floor when she jumped off the bed in the morning. He was always waiting at the bottom of the stairs, and I'd see his wagging tail disappear into the kitchen as I got to the top step. In the kitchen he'd wait to get his head patted before he went outside, and of course there was the thumping, thumping tail.

In the evening after we all had snacks Rasa and Kundun would play in the kitchen. This mainly consisted of them facing each other with bodies poised and tails wagging. Rasa would hit Kundun on the side of his head with the side of her head. She would do this several times. Kundun would playfully snap his teeth. Then Rasa would spread her front legs with her body lowered and quickly move side to side like a football fake-out tactic. It always made me laugh. I can tell that Rasa really misses this, so I begin to try to play with her. At first she is confused about what I am doing and I have to be careful when she becomes confused because she will attack Tara under this circumstance. I try to copy the little gestures they would do with each other and after several tries Rasa gets it. So we now play in the kitchen after snacks, and it seems to lift her spirits, or maybe I look so silly she is laughing.

Every night after Rasa and Tara are on my bed I go back to my bedroom door and look out over the balcony. "Good night Kundun. You have sweet dreams. I love you. We all miss you. You guard the downstairs, okay? But you can come upstairs if you want to. Ganesha's helper—wow, I'm impressed Buddy Boy."

I never leave one dog home alone, so when one dog needs to go somewhere we all go. I begin to realize that Tara is losing her hearing fairly rapidly. One day she cannot hear me from where I sit at my end of the table to her bed at the other end. I adjust how we communicate. Many times I have to walk up to her and touch her in bed to let her know that we're having snacks. I give her visual signals like hold up the container of supplements that I keep in the refrigerator when it's time to go in the laundry room for breakfast. Sometimes I clap to get her attention. Then I realize that I am making a point of calling Tara but I am not also calling Rasa. She stays in her bed feeling rejected. I now call them both. This makes Rasa so happy. I am amazed at how the subtleties have such an importance as they age. I didn't think Rasa and Tara knew which name was which for most of their lives.

Laura leaves a message on my voicemail, "I'm sorry I've taken so long to communicate. I arrived in New York today and received an e-mail that Kay died yesterday."

I cry at the news. I hate cancer. Before leaving after Thanksgiving I sent Kay flowers. The card said, "We love you! Rasa, Tara, Kundun, and Louise." Laura told me then that Kay had been given two weeks to two months. Kay lived one month. I wonder what will happen to her horse and her dogs. I think of our conversation after Kundun died.

Kay told me, "I always wanted to learn to ride a horse, so I just bought one! He is at a stable down the road. I'm taking lessons. He is a very powerful horse but with me he is gentle."

"Oh Kay, what a wonderful adventure to do this! Aren't horses incredible beings?" I think of how many people have a dream and don't realize it, or on the other hand, how many people have a dream and realize it with the threat of terminal cancer. I simultaneously ache for people who don't take the leap to actualize a lifelong dream before dying, or like Kay who actualize it at the last minute.

"I created a trust fund for my dogs," Kay adds.

"I'm scared for you Kay."

"I'm scared too."

We say goodbye.

At night I tell Kundun, "Go see Kay."

I follow the paradigm of do it before they die, and order two large cushy Orvis beds for the kitchen. I also call the fancy pet shop in Santa Fe, Teca Tu, and order two black leather collars with turquoise color stones for them for Christmas. I try to follow Kundun's directive, "Smile, be happy." He lived a happy enthusiastic life no matter what. I'm trying to elevate myself to that level.

38

Christmas this year is sabotaged by the closing paperwork for the sale of the big land and five days of non-stop rain. The day of closing it snowed two feet at the ranch. I am so happy that I don't have to be the one to get the road plowed again. I decorate my little silver fake tree for the kitchen counter and that is all I decide to do this year. While I am taking the decorations for it out of the decoration trunk in the garage I see something wrapped in tissue. I unwrap it and there is Kundun's paw print in white plaster with red and green glitter around the circular edge. Kay made this last year when Kundun stayed with her for the week of Christmas. It never occurred to me then that he wouldn't be with us this year for the holidays or ever again.

Now, they are both gone. After I decorate the little tree with tiny glass icicles and red glass berries, I place the paw print at the base of the tree to remind myself of impermanence. I give thanks that Kundun was part of my life for eleven years, and that we finally found Kay for a happy boarding experience during Kundun's older age where he could have friends to play with in a loving environment.

I stop by Noah's Apocathery where owner, Bea, has a small altar for Kay. There is a photograph of Kay with her dogs together with Bea in front of her natural pet shop. There is a candle, a leather dog leash, and a book to sign. I write, "Kundun loved Kay and Kay loved Kundun. I am certain he was waiting for her on the other side. Rasa and Tara will miss you. Me too. Love, Louise."

I wonder where Kay's dogs are now. Laura has told me they are difficult dogs. I think about Rasa and Tara. They are difficult dogs. I can't die before they do. No one will want them. No one will want their vet bills.

The holidays are quiet. My son and his family are in Santa Fe with his wife's family for Christmas. Cassidy wants to celebrate Christmas at her new home with Alex. She is pregnant now. After all of the expensive procedures with the fertility doctor, who finally told her to look for an egg donor—she got pregnant the low tech way. Three days after Christmas an ultrasound reveals a heartbeat, and of course we are all happy. Rasa will get to smell a baby.

I decide to do something dramatically different and go to Suzanne's for an early New Year's Eve dinner. When I lived in Santa Fe I would go to my zendo to celebrate the arrival of the new year with our one hour before midnight meditation and the ringing of one hundred and eight bells at midnight. After I moved to the ranch I holed up in the cabin with snow whirling quietly except for 1999. That year I carried firewood up the steep trail to the cave trip after trip four or five pieces at a time until I had a stack of firewood in the cave. At eleven I took my bottle of Crystal champagne and a champagne glass, bundled up like an Eskimo, and with Kabuki, my Akita, and Rasa and Tara now one year old, plus my two cats, Pecos and Cimarron, we all paraded up to the cave in the dark with a Coleman lantern lighting the way. I got a roaring fire started, popped the champagne cork, sat back in my log chair and toasted the arrival of the millennium. I could hear fireworks in the far distance while dogs ran in circles crashing through the ponderosas, firs and Gamble oaks on the steep canyon wall chasing rabbits, shadows, and panting in ecstasy from the excitement of a midnight run. I contemplated the ancient Anazazi who stayed in this cave one and two millenniums ago with their furs and fires. I headed back to the house and my warm bed with dogs and cats racing each other to the door.

Kundun tumbled into our lives three days later.

On January second I go to the stable. It is pouring rain. In the past I would've traded days—stayed home the rainy day and gone the next day. However, today I can't wait to experience the stable under the new management which began yesterday. As I drive past the large barn where Natasha kept her horses, I notice that it looks very empty. I can hear the words, "You are never allowed to walk in this barn. You are not allowed to ride your horse on the road behind the corrals in this barn." Of course, those will be two of the first things I do now.

I park and walk up to Genji's stall. "Geeeennnnnjiiii," I whinny. Genji whinnies back, comes up to say hello and eat a piece of carrot. The owner of the mare in the next stall is here and tells me she just turned her horse out in the small covered arena and that the new managers said we can do this in bad weather. I immediately put Genji's halter on and we walk through a blowing torrent of rain to the arena. Genji hasn't had a turnout for several weeks. He runs, kicks, bucks and lets out the energy from days and days of rain and mud in the turnout pens. Well, this is an incredible improvement!

I stop at the large covered arena to say hello to Kimberly and Charles. We discuss the rubber mats in the corrals for the horses in Genji's barn.

Kimberly, tall, slender with long blond hair states, "I was told the boarders own the mats in those corrals."

I add, "And I just found that out today. I've been here one and one-half years and no one ever told me this. Genji has a terrible thrush problem and right now he is ankle deep in mud while he eats his hay. They used to feed the horses in our barn in the stall feeders when it rains. For some reason they aren't doing that now."

"There are things about that barn that I don't understand."

I laugh, "Well if you and your horse were in training then you and your horse got special treatment. Genji is the only horse in that barn that wasn't in training."

"That's not how it is now," Kimberly announces.

I became damp and chilled in the rain at the stable which is now a cold I am fighting. I take Rasa and Tara with me when I return a week later. They need an outing and I don't feel well enough to ride. There is a lot going on at the stable and rumors are rampant. The mare in the stall next to Genji is moving to the large barn behind this barn. Her owner will be training with a different dressage trainer. Baeke, the Fresian, will be moving to the Santa Inez Valley with Natasha. The gelding in the stall on Genji's other side is leaving as well. This empties the barn.

I groom Genji, clean his hooves and put him back in his stall. I give him his apples and carrots. Then I take the book, "Seabisquit," out of my car. I stand in his stall door and read to him. I read about a race. I try to make the imagery strong so he will see it. Genji stands right there while I read. He keeps touching the back of the book with his nose then jumping back. I keep reading trying not to laugh. This is a serious race and Genji was serious about my reading to him. I say, "Genji, this is a book and I'm reading to you like you wanted me to." I am amazed that he is totally engaged in this. He isn't leaving the stall. He isn't moving. I finish reading, say goodbye and leave. I definitely will continue our reading sessions with more races, because I think anything else in the story will be boring to him.

On the drive home I think of Genji saying that this stable is "at Heaven's gate," and I simply cannot move him because things are shifting and changing with the new management. I want to give it a chance to settle down. Natasha was hands on aggressively micro-managing everything—yelling from a distance and roaring around on her ATV outfitted with a western-style wool, stripe saddle blanket. She stood up hair flying behind her as she traversed the stable from one end to the other at full speed leaving a trail of dust. The new managers are hands off, consider the employees adults who don't need micro-managing. This has many horse owners in fear. They tell me the blankets aren't being taken off when the day warms up, the supplements aren't being fed. I don't shear and blanket Genji in the winter. He is a wooly looking pony until he sheds in the spring. We all count our individual week's supplement bags to insure that they are being fed. Often they aren't, however now there is a discrepancy between owners and employees about the situation.

The main thing I have noticed in one week is the quiet and calm. The frenetic energy is gone and I like that. The place looks half empty with the sheep, cows, and mules gone plus several large corrals and one barn emptied of horses. I had no idea so many of the animals here belonged to the management.

When I get home I call Laura to tell her about our reading experience, "Now we have to make an appointment to talk to Genji because I'm curious to find out if this worked for him. When Genji asked me to read aloud so that the other horses can hear the story also, how does that work?"

"Do you know how dogs watch TV, except they aren't necessarily looking at the TV? They can watch it through your mind."

"Wow, so the other horses can see the story through Genji's mind?"

"Yes."

"It's wild. Bea told me that Kay's son is taking her two dogs back to Sweden with him."

"I can't make her memorial, I have a radio interview."

"I'm not going. I feel too sick."

39

"Tara, how did you enjoy going to the stable today?"

"I feel freedom to go there. Nothing scares me there. I think Genji needs more bedding. Kundun watches us there. Mom isn't drinking enough tea. When she drinks more tea, she feels better. It makes her lower bones not hurt."

"What do you mean by lower bones?" Laura asks. "She means your hips," Laura explains to me. "Tara is really talking a lot today."

"Tara is much more confident since Kundun died. She is playful and silly like she was before Jake kicked her. For the first time in five years I feel like I have my dog back. I've taken her off Rescue Remedy."

"Kundun gave me strength," Tara responds.

I wonder at the miracle of such a gift bestowed by our angel, Kundun. I also have Dr. Alice to thank for putting Tara on a new product that is made for people called Vitality. She has us all on it including me.

"The Feng Shui woman wants to plant a tree in front of the front door," Tara states.

"This is actually the back door because we never use the front door," I explain.

"The trees don't want any more trees planted here," Tara adds.

"Did the trees tell you?" Laura asks.

"Yes."

"How long have you been talking to trees?"

"I always have. Kundun talks to coyotes. I don't"

After Tara's lengthy dialogue, Rasa speaks up, "The Feng Shui lady kept saying to herself, 'These are interesting dogs.' I was listening to see what else she thought, but she kept saying, 'These are interesting dogs.'"

Tara says, "I want a little more food. I am still hungry after I eat. A capsule with oil in it in a brown bottle makes hips feel better."

Tara is a very fit dog. She has muscle definition all over her body including her back. I think she looks perfect, however I don't want her to feel hungry. I cannot remember these capsules, but I think Kundun took them at some point.

Rasa goes back to my question about going to the stable today, "The stable is mine, the dogs are gone. I want to go every day. I want to go to the water. I can smell water."

"I'm trying to take them with me frequently while it is still cool, and to take them on more walks to different places. There is a creek at the stable, Rasa must smell that."

"When I go with Mom my head doesn't go in circles. I realize the world is bigger than us. There is the spirit world also. That elephant man isn't as nice to me as Kundun."

I ask Tara, "What does he do?"

"He twirls his hand and tells me to jump over it. He says I can do it."

I look at Laura, and the image of Ganesha doing this strikes me as hilarious. I can't help myself and I burst into laughter hoping I'm not hurting Tara's feelings.

"Rasa, do you talk to the elephant man?" I ask curiously.

"No, a lady holding a flower talks to me."

Laura looks at me and asks, "Who is that?"

"The bodhisattva, Tara, or Kuan Yin. They each hold a lotus."

Rasa states, "Kay is sorry that she died and is worried about her dogs. I can look at people and see if cancer gets better or worse. With Kay it was worse, with Mom—better."

"Do you have cancer?" Laura asks with a surprised look.

"Yes, ongoing skin cancer on my face. Do they have any questions for me?"

Rasa asks, "Do you have your own star? When I go outside at night, I think there is a star that shines just for me." She adds, "Cassidy should chew on roots, they will make her feel better."

I can't answer Rasa's question, but it is something beautiful to ponder. I do pass her wisdom about chewing on roots to Cassidy, who has morning sickness all day and night.

Tara asks, "When you are a dog with a pregnant person are you happy or scared?"

"Both," Laura answers.

"Crush is scared of wheels. He wonders if his bed will move. He needs to come for a visit."

Laura looks at the clock and says, "It's time for me to go."

"Oh, we forgot to talk to Kundun!"

"I went with you to the stable today. I think you should sleep on your left side. I helped you find the Feng Shui lady. Don't plant a tree! I go upstairs a lot. I sit on your right when you mediate. Meditate longer!"

"Do you have a question for Kundun?" Laura asks.

After what seems like a long pause, I ask, "Do you have advice for me about the book?"

"Can you open the book with chanting? You need to move the first chapter into the book further."

Laura leaves and I reflect on everything Kundun said. I have been doing short meditations, my theory being to get on my cushion even if it's for ten minutes. Obviously this doesn't cut it. I cannot underestimate the significance of Kundun sitting on my right while I meditate, because four feet to my right is a bronze statue of Ganesha. It is a huge statue of him sitting on a pillowed bench with an umbrella over his head and the wheel of dharma behind his head. In his four hands he holds a hatchet to cut through the bondage created by desire, a sweet fruit symbolizing the sweetness of true knowledge, the end of his broken off tusk, and an object that looks like a weapon and is probably for cutting through delusion. On a little stool below his feet is a rat, his vehicle. The rat symbolizes the demon of vanity. Around his waist is a cobra in reference to his father, Lord Shiva. The snakes represent tamed passions. Embossed on his trunk between his eyes is a trident which symbolizes the balance of the forces of creation, preservation and destruction. Ganesha creates the faith to remove all obstacles, removing doubts and therefore pointing out the spiritual side of everything.

40

Genji whinnies when I arrive in my car. I always park in front of his stall under the pepper tree. I walk across the lush green lawn between the parking area and his barn to give him a piece of carrot. Laura arrives as I am getting his halter.

"Hello Laura, how are you?"

She steps into the stall, "Genji how are you feeling with all of the horses gone now?"

Every horse has left Genji's barn now, the last two yesterday. A tall, bay Thoroughbred mare moved in to the empty end stall a week ago. She had been in a corral.

"I might want to move to a different barn. The wind blows through my barn and rattles everything."

"Do you want to look at another barn?" Laura asks.

"Let's walk over to the big barn there," I motion.

Laura, Genji, and I walk to the big barn behind Genji's barn. It has an aisle with six stalls and corrals on each side. There are two sets of cross-ties and two tack rooms in the center. The barn is almost empty at this point.

"Are these stalls empty?"

"If the stall doors have blankets hanging on them they are occupied. Some of the horses are having turnouts."

"Here is an empty stall. Do you want to look at this one Genji?"

We all walk into the stall, then out the other side into the corral. "See how his barn has trees in front and how it is in the shade now? It really is the nicest barn."

"Do you like the view from here Genji?"

Genji doesn't answer Laura's question. Instead he asks me a question, "Are there exercises you can do for your back?"

My back ached a little after our ride yesterday and Genji is apparently aware of this. "Yes, there are, but I have no energy to do them because I am sick with bronchitis."

We turn around and walk back out of the stall, down the aisle and over to the green grass growing next to the small covered arena. On the way Genji asks, "Can we have Feng Shui done on the barn?"

This is probably a good idea. I'd never thought about doing Feng Shui on a barn. Laura tells me some people do it. Genji is busy grazing while we talk.

"Tell us a story. You have good stories," I say.

"The horses all went to different places and at first we were talking to each other about where they each were. Now we are not talking so much. One horse thought he was leaving to go to a show, and he never came back to the stable again. One horse thought he was going to be given away."

This is not one of Genji's light-hearted stories.

"What does Genji know about the little horse in that barn over there? The little horse that starved and died? I was told that I was not allowed to ever set foot in the big barn over there." I motion toward the barn Natasha used that is attached to the large covered arena. "So, the first thing I did after Natasha left was to walk through that barn. I had Rasa and Tara with me. We went in through the door on that end, walked to the other end, noted that two horses were in two of the stalls with corrals, then turned around to walk back out. I caught movement out of the corner of my right eye. I turned and looked into a dark stall. Since it is in the middle of the barn, it has no corral because the arena is directly behind the stalls on that side of the barn. I was horrified to see a small dark brown horse that was a skeleton with hide. The horse touched my hand with its soft nose. This horse was being hidden in this dark stall. I thought of a photograph of a rescued horse in an animal rescue newsletter. The vet said that horse would have died in two more days. This is how this horse looks, maybe worse. I debated for hours whether I should call the Humane Society to report it. I did not. They had been out there previously, but I didn't feel that they got a straight story and nothing was done."

It took me two weeks to get back to that stall. The horse was gone. I could see where the horse had laid on the stall floor, and had been dragged out. It's illegal to bury a euthanized horse in California because of the toxins from the euthanasia which can get into the groundwater. So if a horse dies some other way, it can be buried and not hauled away.

Genji responds, "They fed him one flake of hay a day and let him die. His mom paid money every month to take care of him."

Laura turns away and I can see that she is fighting tears, "I am outraged."

"If I ever see a horse like that here again, I'll report it. This is their horse retirement program. They put the horses out on pasture with no hay. The younger horses do fairly well, but not the older ones."

I change the subject, "How does Genji feel about staying here? I just want him to be happy."

"I think many horses will come to the stable, ponies also. There will be nice people, a trainer."

"Wow, how do you know that?"

"Kundun is working on it."

"What does Kundun have to say?"

"I am helping the Feng Shui lady. I am having fun here. I like being here."

"I wish Maia liked it there," Laura says.

"Maia doesn't like it?"

"No, she wants to come back soon."

Maia is Laura's wolf-dog that died last August.

"What happened to Kay's horse?"

"There is a woman at the stable who helped Kay a lot with her horse. She didn't have the money to buy a nice horse. Kay gave him to her."

"That was generous." I think of what a wonderful part of Kay's life that horse became, and now he has another loving owner. If only every horse had a similar story.

41

Tara's ability to hear is slipping away rapidly. I either need to clap or go to her bed and touch her so that she knows it is snack time, or dinner time, or we are going to the car. Because Rasa and Tara spent our hikes running like crazy hounds through the dense oak and pines, I didn't teach many hand signals to them. I had a little black plastic whistle, my own pathetic not very loud whistle, and my voice. Because I spent most of our hikes looking at their hind ends as they ran ahead with noses to the ground and tails wagging, I began to try to identify which dog was which by any differences I could determine. This is when I eventually realized that Tara has a perfect heart-shaped anus. An anus is not a body part that I ever considered remotely cute, however Tara's heart-anus ranks as adorable and unique no matter what.

Tara lies on her bed, the new cushy Orvis bagel bed, looking out the kitchen French glass doors for coyotes, or she sleeps. I realize she probably no longer hears the music I play in the morning.

So, when Laura comes to visit, my first question is, "How are you doing Tara with not being able to hear?"

"I'm starting to like Lisa. I like to be at home rather than at the kennel. The kennel is too stressful—I poop all the time. My ears feel clogged. It doesn't hurt. It's an empty feeling."

"You heard me come in the door," Laura states.

"I sensed you like the wind. My right ear is worse. I hear doors in the wind. I want to go to Cynthia's, but I can't hear the tuning fork."

Rasa comes downstairs from my office and joins the conversation. "The Feng Shui lady told the trees to shut-up and behave. She thinks everything is wrong here except me, Tara, and Mom. Lisa likes us a lot. She brought me a tasty treat. Sometimes I was at Mom's retreat and meditated with her. I am better than Lama Norbu! I have a happy friend in my head that helps me feel brave when I'm not."

I am surprised by Rasa's comment about not feeling brave. "When aren't you feeling brave?"

"When Lisa said, 'It was great seeing you guys,' and left. I knew Mom wasn't coming home until the next day."

Laura looks horrified.

"I left my retreat at the Vajrapani Institute and drove south to Big Sur. When I arrived at my hotel I checked my cell phone to see if it was charged and it wasn't. However my phone alerted me to two messages. My daughter had called to wish me Happy Birthday, and Lisa had called, thankfully, indicating that I would be home by now. I frantically called her at four-thirty and she went to the house to feed them. I do not know why she was so confused, but thank heavens she left a message and that I checked messages."

Rasa adds, "I want a long walk."

"Rasa attacked Tara at the stable, why did she do that?"

"I don't have anything to say. I think I did the wrong thing."

"Tara was tough and fought Rasa. It sounded like they were killing each other. I had them on leashes and in the process of trying to separate them I blocked Rasa with my leg and have a major bruise on the side of my knee."

Tara says, "You have to be bold."

"It wasn't that bad," Rasa adds.

"Let's talk to Kundun," Laura suggests.

"I'm spending a lot of time at the big land. I'm in Whippet form to move fast. The new owners are moving things on the trails and I'm trying to stop it."

I look at Laura, "I dismantled everything except for a few things before I left. The trails are all covered with snow right now. He must mean the Zen garden. They are building a master bathroom in that area."

I remember how the Zen garden was originally the dog yard. It is where Rasa and Tara were assaulted by workmen. It was so unbearable to even look at the place where my precious puppies were physically and emotionally terrorized that I decided to remove the metal gate and wire fence on one side to create a beautiful place to sit and reflect. I enjoyed this project and Jake worked diligently to bring my ideas to fruition. We attached reed fencing to the wire on the north and south sides. The east side is open to the creek with a tall ponderosa pine and a cedar shading the area much of the day. Red-osier dogwood and Nanking cherry bushes were planted as well as lavender and decorative grasses. I found a granite basin with a bamboo water spout for a fountain. All of the iris that had been planted along the creek, and which had over almost twenty years multiplied, become dwarfed, and reverted to the original wild iris color of deep blue were dug up and relocated into this garden. I had enjoyed them along the creek, however a huge flood had ripped out many of them, so I wanted to save the remainder. I found two live cedar trees with forked tops and had Jake cut those down for the entrance gate. A third curved cedar branch rested between the two forked trees, which I thought looked perfect. With the finishing touches of a bench, and a cobblestone path to the bench, my garden was ready to enjoy.

At the end of my walks with Kundun I would bow at the gate, like magic the wind chime would greet me, and I would walk to my bench to enjoy the garden in every season. Kundun, of course, always joined me there. In my mind it is all the way it was when I lived there. I gave the buyers the idea to make the master bedroom larger by tearing out the existing bathroom and going through the log wall to add a bathroom where the Zen garden is.

Kundun continues, "I am with you when you meditate. Radiate up, not out. If you radiate out the trees take it. You need to pay attention to the way people and spaces feel. I want to come back as a person to communicate with humans because they are confusing. They don't always say what they are thinking. With dogs it is clear!"

"How do you like Lama Norbu?"

"He is born from my belly and other bellies like mine. He is like the first breath of fresh air after you've been sick. You need a joyful teacher. There isn't enough joy in your life."

"Do you have questions or requests for me?"

"I want my ear unclogged and a long walk also, plus some meat strips." This is Tara's favorite special treat—sautéed stir-fry beef.

"I want a bowl of water with crystals in it," Rasa adds.

"I miss Kundun a lot. I like it when you talk to him," Tara tells us.

"How do you see Kundun?" I ask.

"I see him as a fiery light like what the sun looks like. I tell him to look like his dog-self."

Laura changes the subject. "Let's talk to Kay." Laura closes her eyes and has a similar expression on her face as when she is communicating with

Kundun. She told me in the beginning that she could also communicate with people on the other side.

"Louise has a kind heart, and when she is gone, I look after the dogs. I died too young and I don't want to be here. Everything I loved I left behind. I'm worried about my dogs. They are confused. I spend a lot of time with them."

Laura and I discuss this situation. "Did I tell you that Maia got stuck in a dark box? I think she didn't go high enough when she crossed over. I think Kay has the same problem."

"What about ghosts?"

"They didn't cross over at all. They are still stuck in this realm."

"This is a lot more to contemplate than I ever would have guessed."

42

"Hello Genji, wow you look beautiful! How are you?" Laura, Genji and I move from the barn area to the grass near the turn-out pens.

"What do you want to talk about today?"

"Genji, how did you like the book I read to you about one of Seabisquit's races, and did I do a good job of reading it so you could understand me?"

"We all listened to the story, and later we talked about it. We talked about his passion for running and how none of us feel like we have that much passion about running or about anything."

"I am elated that Genji, that all of them understood me. I tried really hard to have strong visual images. Also, I just saw the Seabisquit movie when it was shown in Ojai a month ago for a fundraiser for the local horse rescue sanctuary. So the images are fresh in my mind."

"But Genji, you have a passion for going riding."

"Not like that."

"On the trails?"

"I have passion for my mom."

"What does the old horse next to you say?"

"The people who were taking care of him weren't feeding him enough, but now he is happy to be in the barn."

I explain to Laura, "He is old—thirty something, and apparently well-loved because at some point he had surgery and has a partially titanium leg. He is that horse right there in the turn-out pen."

Laura looks over at the roan colored, rangy, white faced former cow pony.

"He is thin and bony, but looks much better than the first day I saw him a few weeks earlier. I think he is one of the pasture horses. The management is giving every boarder who stayed and who has a horse in a stall a ten percent discount for the rest of the year. You can see from here how nice it looks now.

They moved out that ugly old trailer, are rebuilding the wash racks, and look, all of those pens that were there are gone now."

"What was in those pens," Laura asks.

"Cows, sheep, the former manager's horses. It doesn't look like a rodeo facility anymore."

"We are all proud to be here," Genji says. "The difficult horses are all gone."

"But the stable needs more horses to have a viable business."

"They want people to talk about it, so there will be rumors about what a wonderful place it is."

Laura and I both laugh.

Genji asks, "Did any horses die in the tsunami?"

"How does he know about the tsunami?"

"All of the animals know about the tsunami," Laura responds.

"I don't know Genji," I answer. "There was farmland in the area, but there is nothing on the news about animals. Maybe there weren't horses."

"People all over the world love and have horses," Genji states emphatically.

"You're right, so perhaps horses died."

"I watched a video on You Tube filmed by Japanese people. They were speaking Japanese so I couldn't understand them," Laura tells us. "There were two dogs, one was a Brittany Spaniel. The other dog looked dead. The Spaniel sat next to the other dog then leaned on him. Next the Spaniel started to paw his head. Then the other dog feebly lifted up his head."

"He was trying to get help," I exclaim amazed.

"I talked to the Spaniel. His mom and dad were communicating from Heaven, so he knew they had died, but he didn't know what had happened to the children. There is a shark feeding frenzy in the ocean, but they are getting sick because they aren't used to that kind of food. There is radioactive water leaking into the ocean that they aren't admitting."

"When my family was here we went kayaking in the Santa Barbara Harbor."

"You are brave, I would never have done that," Laura remarks.

"The tsunami was Thursday. The beaches and harbors were closed in California Friday. The kayaking trips were cancelled, so we went Saturday. We had the wildest experience with the surges from after-shocks. We were having lunch on a little beach at the base of the harbor sea wall. All of a sudden a surge of water lifted up one of the kayaks, and the beach began to disappear. We were grabbing life vests that were floating and stacking up the kayaks, moving the lunch table closer to the rocks. A whirlpool formed in front of us. It was a miniature real time experience in exactly what happened on a much larger scale in Japan. We had three surges during our lunch. When we paddled out to the buoy in an unusually calm ocean, our guide said, 'There are always sea lions and harbor seals on the buoy.' There were none"

"I'll have to talk to the sea animals," Laura reflects.

"The day we met with Rasa and Tara, Bhakti died. I wonder why Kundun didn't tell us. He died several hours earlier."

Laura checks in with Kundun and they have a lengthy conversation. Genji is grazing and slowly moving around to the backside of the turn-out pens.

"Kundun said that he didn't tell us because time is different there. I said, 'I don't buy that.' Then he said that it takes time to make the transition. I said, 'I don't buy that.' Then Kundun explained that he couldn't tell us or you would have known before Will and Elizabeth did."

"Did Bhakti feel that he died with people who love him? He had a very bad night before he died, and was euthanized."

Bhakti tells us, "I was very sick, but there was a comforting warmth like a blanket wrapped around me that made me feel peaceful. I died peacefully. It didn't matter if they were with me or not because I had the blanket."

"Angels around his aura," Laura explains.

"Is he with you, Kundun?" I wonder.

"Bhakti slept for three days on a round blue bed. Then we ran together across the land."

"It's not the big land. He is showing me somewhere else."

Bhakti speaks again, "Thank you for talking to me, it helped me a lot."

"Do you mean when I was in Santa Fe last year?"

Laura nods her head yes.

I reflect on those last special moments we had together.

Genji is pulling me along now and we have circumambulated the turn out pens. Genji suddenly jumps and in the process kicks me in the leg above the ankle. "He has never done this, what is happening?"

A mare gallops down the side of her turn out pen with her head lowered and crashes her forehead into the center metal rail at the end of the pen. Laura takes Genji's lead rope, gets him to stand next to the turn out pen fence and talks to him.

"When something scares you remember this: lick your tongue, chew, blink your eyes then think about it before you react." She goes over this several times then adds, "or you will hurt your mom."

Back at the barn and tied to the saddling rail, Genji offers, "When one horse gets upset, we all get upset. Let's go for a ride!"

In the afternoon Tara has an appointment with Dr. Nicci. The coughing has stopped and I conclude that it could be temperature related. The nights have warmed up. The house isn't so cold now, and I am able to open the bedroom window for fresh air while we sleep. Tara has another problem. She is moving her right hind leg strangely. She is picking it up too high when she walks. She also seems to have trouble getting up into a sitting position and from there to standing up. I've been observing this for a week now and am concerned. Her leg seems feeble.

Dr. Nicci suggests X-rays of her lower back mainly because that is where her cancer tumor was removed on the right side of her spine. She places Tara's previous chest X-rays up on the lighted X-ray viewing board.

"I was hoping that her chest X-rays would also have included this area of her lower back, but you can see how differently we have to do an X-ray for soft tissue than for bones." She points to the lungs which are in detail, and then to the vertebrae which are light and almost blurry.

So, I schedule Tara for X-rays and Rasa for a teeth cleaning, which should have been done in November, but I couldn't afford it right before the holidays.

43

On Tuesday Tara has her lower back X-rays. Her hind right leg is unsteady and she loses her balance on this leg plus stumbles frequently. I notice this once I begin to watch her when she is outside. Dr. Jill shows me the X-rays.

"You can see on this last vertebra how it has clear defined edges. There is no arthritis here. You can see how the other vertebrae have less defined edges and jagged looking places. That is the arthritis. Our greatest concern is this last vertebra before the tail. When this gets arthritis it causes many problems." Dr. Jill conveys with the expression on her face that there is nothing you can do at that point.

I now understand Tara's mobility issues. I realize this will get worse and worse. After Kundun's experience with anti-inflammatory drugs, I decide they are not an option. Tara is placed on a muscle relaxer and a drug that helps the nerves, Gabapentin.

"Are there any side effects with the Gabapentin?"

"Personality change."

"I'll watch her carefully."

On Thursday I go to the stable. Thursday is the last day of March. When you board a horse, you pay the board for the month in advance. When you decide to leave, the boarding contract generally requests a thirty day notice. So when horses move it is usually on the last day of the month. As I pull into the stable gate I see two large horse trailers parked by the large barn. As I park at the edge of the grass in front of Genji's stall I see a two-horse trailer unloading in front of the row of corrals west of his barn. From the large barn come whinnies of horses in a new place.

All of this ebullience makes Genji excited and nervous. When Kimberly and Charles drive by while I am grooming him, I say, "It looks like some new horses have arrived."

"We have twenty-one horses moving in today. Fourteen are in the big barn and the other seven are scattered around. One is in your barn. The fourteen are in between stables, but we hope they stay here."

"Wonderful, congratulations!"

And so Genji's and Kundun's prophecy that lots of horses are coming to live here is fulfilled. I begin our ride in the large covered arena. The weather has gone from cold to hot in just a few days. Then being curious about the new horses, I ride behind the corrals of the big barn to have a look. They appear to be quarter horses, very nice quarter horses. There are two palominos.

Since it is so hot today, I decide to ride on the trail past the hay barn that goes up to a tower for electrical lines that cross the valley. We are treated to a meadow of green grass so thick the ground disappears beneath it. "Remember the meadow in Pecos, Genji? It was like this except it was full of flowers—Indian paintbrush, lupine, yarrow." Picnic tables have been set up under one of the oak trees. It looks like a park in this area now after last year's grading, tree trimming and deadwood removal. Before the rainy season it was all loose dirt baking in the heat.

A creek flows below the trail that is located on the north facing side of the mountain. Beautiful huge live oaks, sycamores and locust trees provide a shady canopy until the top which is scrubby chaparral. The trail took a beating in the last ferocious storm of wind and rain. The creek side edge is collapsing down toward the creek in places. The uphill side has collapsed down onto the trail in places. A tree has fallen across the trail, but there is room to ride around it by going off the trail. Wild pigs have had a rooting frenzy and I notice deer tracks as well as the pig tracks. It is a good trail for Genji to get back in shape after his winter rest. It is fairly flat with a gradual incline to a certain point. Then it becomes steep from there to the tower. The hot air rises up the steep mountain on the south side and hits like a furnace blast when you reach the ridge at the top. Red tail hawks cruise the thermals here. There is an eight foot wide roadway that drops straight down on both sides where it traverses a narrow ridge. It is frightening to ride from the top of the trail to the tower, especially on a nervous horse. After the adrenaline rush for about fifty feet, the view of the Canada Larga valley extending five miles to the west is breathtaking.

The west end of the valley came out of the lands that belonged to the San Buenaventura Mission. Following the Mexican independence from Spain, then Governor Juan Batista Alvarado granted six thousand, six hundred and fifty-nine acres to Joaquina Alvarado de Moraga, whose late husband was a distinguished soldier of Spanish California. She received possession in 1847 one year after California became part of the United States. Remnants of the mission aqueduct which carried water from the San Antonio Creek to the San Buenaventura Mission are still visible by the road at the entrance to the valley. Over one hundred and fifty years later this is still all open privately owned land used for cattle ranching.

We have a great ride. Genji is willing to go to the top, but I end our ride where the shade stops. He is drenched in sweat from the heat, from still not having shed the remainder of his winter coat, and from the exertion of a steep hill, which he never does ploddingly. We finish back at the barn with a hosing off and more grooming.

As I drive out yet another horse trailer pulls up to the large barn. It is a very fancy rig and on the side in ornate lettering it says, "Performance Horses." I smile as I realize I was in on a big tip and how it never occurred to me that Genji and Kundun meant that lots of horses would all arrive on the same day. The mystery and wonder of it fills my heart with laughter.

44

When Laura walks into the kitchen she exclaims, "Oh you have rearranged it!"

"Yes, I pulled the table out more and now have Tara's bed in this corner where I can see her from my chair. Now that she is so deaf, I can get her attention easier. I was originally trying to get her out of a traffic zone and have the table more accessible while my son and his family visited in March."

"I'm going to move this chair to the end of the table so I can see Tara. What do you want to ask them?"

"Tara, are you getting enough to eat?"

"I want more of the food in a bag and more kibble. I like the chews."

"The food in a bag is the chicken and pumpkin soup. I pour that over the kibble now that she is off the raw diet. See how her ribs stick out? I worry about her."

"I think she looks great."

"I want more to eat too," Rasa adds.

"How was Lisa?" Laura asks.

"She got us right, Tara answers, but the light is too bright at night."

I explain, "I have her leave the light on over the stove. It's on a dimmer, but now that it's light outside later, I guess it's hard to tell how dim it is."

"Without Kundun I'm really lonely when you leave. Lisa doesn't spend a lot of time talking to us like you do," Rasa tells us sadly.

"They are going to Kay's former and now revived kennel in three weeks when I go to my nephew's college graduation in Dallas."

"Will I sleep on a towel?" Tara asks.

I look at Laura with a questioning frown.

"I don't think they sleep on towels there."

"I'll take a bed for you, Tara."

"I've visited Kay's house with my mind and it seems empty," states Rasa.

"I wonder if they moved out a lot of Kay's things," Laura responds.

"When Kundun was alive I thought he would live longer than me, now I see him jumping over the fence and I am envious," says Rasa.

I think of Kundun jumping over the dog yard fence at the big land. He had a broad pit bull chest, but long legs and was surprisingly agile and fast for his build.

"Cassidy's baby is going to be wild!" Tara exclaims.

"She is calling him a coyote because he has a sense of humor," I laugh.

Laura thinks maybe Tara is confused by this, "He won't be a wild animal."

"Have Rasa and Tara talked to the coyotes? Where are they? We haven't seen them for a long time."

"A man on the hill shot them because they killed his cat."

"How do you know, Tara?"

"A jay told me. The jay said the coyotes are dying and asked if Mom knows a doctor who can help them? I told the jay that she knows a doctor, but not one that can help coyotes."

"Did Rasa and Tara know that the oak tree was going to fall over?"

I reflect on the storm, the non-stop down rush of rain for days, and what seemed like hurricane force wind. Rasa and Tara did not want to go outside for a potty break. I put on my rain jacket and grabbed my bright red umbrella. We all went out the kitchen door. I walked down the several steps into the center of the cobblestone courtyard. "Come on let's go potty." They stood on the top step and looked at me with big eyes and wouldn't move. We went back in the house. I went upstairs to watch the huge oaks on the other side of the house as they blew back and forth. I was worried about my car. I returned to the kitchen a few minutes later and the entire courtyard was filled with the oak tree that had fallen over. I had been standing in a direct line with the tree trunk.

"I felt a rumbling under the house. The trees screamed, 'Get her out of there!'" Tara responds.

"I think Kundun had something to do with the tree not falling on Mom," Rasa adds. "Genji has lots of friends now. Before they came to the stable, the horses were treated well so they have nice things to talk about."

"Shall we talk to Kundun?" Laura closes her eyes as she contacts Kundun.

"I've been exploring. I discovered sea shells. You should go somewhere you can find sea shells. A lot of animals drowned in the tsunami. I helped them swim out to get to Heaven."

"What is Bhakti doing?"

"He is looking after Alan. He is smoothing out the energy field so Alan can disappear easier."

After Bhakti died, every night when I'd talk to Kundun, I'd tell Bhakti, "Take care of Alan, Bhakti, he needs you now. Be his angel."

I'm fascinated by how the dog spirits or angel dogs immediately find their responsibility or mission to help still earthbound beings, so I look at Laura and inquire, "Do you hear this..." The rest of my sentence is unnecessary. Laura nods her head affirmatively and we are both quiet in the mystery of it.

"Kundun is in a very joyful place," Laura adds.

"Are you still helping Ganesha?"

"Yes, I'm helping a little girl."

"She looks three or four years old. Is she in your family?"

"There is no one that young in my family. I miss you Kundun."

"The trees love Mom," he responds.

"Every night when I go out with Rasa and Tara I say, 'Goodnight oak people. Thank you for being here.' I think it's important to express appreciation to all living beings."

"I love you, Mom," Kundun finishes.

"Genji wants his mane unbraided and brushed and you to read to him again," Rasa says.

"I want to walk on the beach," Tara emphatically adds.

"We'll go Monday."

Laura counts out the days for her.

"Do I get more food tonight?" Rasa wants to know.

"Yes!"

The morning following our conversation with Laura I am sitting at the kitchen table drinking my cup of Russian Caravan tea. Tara gets up out of her bed on my left and walks to the water bowl on my right. I watch how she walks because now I have cut her Gabapentin from three pills two times a day to one pill two times a day. After Cynthia said that she was absolutely flat a week ago, I started taking her off it slowly. Tara didn't test for working on anything in her body, and since Cynthia's work is predicated on the body healing itself on a cellular level, this is problematic.

I observe that she is still picking her right hind foot up higher than necessary, and as I am focused on her leg I see a round lump three inches above her hock. I wait until she finishes drinking her water and returns to her bed. I get out of my chair, walk around the table and crouch by her bed. I pet her and my hand goes to the lump. This lump absolutely was not there Sunday when I left for Los Angeles to visit Cassidy for a few days. I call Buena as soon as they open at eight A.M. Dr. Nicci is booked all day. I make an appointment for the following day on Saturday.

Tara's whole body starts shaking the second we walk in the clinic door. We are ushered into a little room to wait for Dr. Nicci. First she looks at Rasa's teeth and is astonished at how fast the plaque has built up on her teeth in two and one-half weeks. She shows me how to brush her teeth and apply the plaque prevention gel. Since Rasa can't chew on bones because they will break her teeth now, her teeth don't stay clean.

Next we talk about Tara's lump. "I cut back on supplements—they are so expensive."

"Don't beat yourself up about that. You brought her in quickly." She aspirates it with a needle and prepares a slide. "I'll be back in a few minutes."

Rasa and Tara nervously rub against my legs. For some reason when we go to Buena I always seem to wear black jeans which become covered with hair. I keep brushing the hair off my pants with my hand and try to keep my mind in the present moment, but I have a bad feeling about this. It grew too fast. It's too close to the original tumor on her back. There is no way to get a three centimeter margin without amputating her leg, which I won't do. After the embolism she can barely support herself to pee. She would simply never try to get up again without her leg. My head swirls with fear, resignation, helplessness, and sorrow. Finally, after what seems like an hour dragging by, Dr. Nicci comes back into the room.

"This does not look good."

"Do you recommend a biopsy?"

"I think she needs to have surgery to remove the lump. We can't get a margin. I'll send in a biopsy."

"You are here Wednesday to Saturday?"

"Yes, let me look at my schedule. I can do it Wednesday. You know the routine. Let me get a proposal for you. I'll meet you in front."

"Okay, I'll put the dogs in the car."

There is only one positive aspect to this. I didn't dream about Wuli. I take Rasa and Tara to the big grass for a quick walk. It is Saturday, it's sunny, and there are people everywhere enjoying the weather—walking, bicycling, picnicking, jogging.

On the drive home I talk to Tara, "I'll get the front porch finished with a gate so you can enjoy going out there. We'll go to Carpenteria to walk on Santa Claus Beach. I won't leave after I go to my nephews' college graduations in May and June. We'll spend our time together while we can. You'll make it to your thirteenth birthday, Tara. I'll ramp up the supplements. We'll keep going to Dr. Alice."

But inside I feel a crushing weight on my heart. Tears fill my eyes, but they don't spill out. I cannot bear the thought of losing my precious Tara, Dolly Girl, Miss Patuti, my crazy loveable Catahoula. Of course I knew this would happen someday, but someday is never now. It is a place in the future that you don't want to look for or find. It's over there somewhere far away.

I am thankful to have some warning unlike with Kundun. However as Dr. Nicci pointed out, although I saw everything happen to him in one week—in dog aging time, it was over one month. So, Tara is approaching her thirteenth birthday in human time—her ninety-first in dog time.

45

Tara's surgery goes well. She has her teeth cleaned while she is under anesthesia. I worry about her all day and am happy when she is home again. She has to be walked on a leash to go outside. For the first couple of days we seem to do this twenty times a day. I keep her in the kitchen the first night, but let her come to bed after that.

I watch Tara in her bed from my chair at the table. The chairs are Adirondak hickory chairs with bright red floral upholstery. They have high backs and mine has hickory arms which catch the threads on the sleeves of various articles of clothing and ruin them. The chairs looked quite fabulous in my log house in New Mexico, but don't really fit in my Mediterranean house style here in California. I keep them because they are comfortable and because the vet bills are endless and I can't afford the wicker chairs I'd like to have. Tara is aging rapidly. When she lies down her ribs and hips protrude, but her belly looks fat. Her facial bones are more pronounced. She sleeps most of the time. Her eyes look sad. Most frightening though is that she is becoming confused and disoriented.

I fix Rasa's and Tara's meals in the laundry room. I used to say, "Okay, its dinner time," and Tara would excitedly bounce and wiggle in the kitchen as I gathered the supplements from the refrigerator, a spoon, and walked into the laundry room. Rasa meanwhile would get one of her toys—froggie, monkey or ducky and chew on it to make the frog repeatedly say ribbit, the duck supposedly quack, but instead it sounds like Penguin in Batman, or the monkey make a monkey sound. Meal times were always animated and festive. In the laundry room I keep the kibble in a plastic container in a deep drawer. Tara always sits on the right of the drawer on a little rug and Rasa on the left on a little rug in front of the sink. I scoop the kibble into their dishes which are on the counter. Their dishes are fabulous ceramic bowls with dots, bones and paw prints painted on them. Rasa's bowl has a blue rim and Tara's bowl has a brown rim. I arbitrarily matched the rims to their eye colors to decide which bowl is which dog's. I take four or five pieces of kibble out of each bowl and say, "Okay this is for Tara," and put it on the rug for a pre-meal treat. Then I say, "Okay this is for Rasa," and put it on her rug. Then I close the drawer and say, "Okay!" Rasa picks up her toy and moves to the rug just outside the laundry room where she eats, and Tara switches from the rug she is on to the rug Rasa just left and turns around to face me while I finish adding the supplements. They invented this routine after we moved here and we've done it ever since two meals a day.

Tara comes in the laundry room but leaves before the treats. I give Rasa her treats and her dinner then go look for Tara. She isn't in the kitchen. I look upstairs in my office, the office bathroom. I begin to panic a little. I look again in the kitchen, the bathroom next to the kitchen and even look in the shower behind the curtain. I look right at the studio door which is closed, and I open it. There is Tara! She must have thought that was the laundry room. She can't hear me, so she pushed the studio door open, went in, and it closed behind her because this door does that.

"Oh Tara there you are! Come this way." I move my hands together with a come toward me motion.

The following day I leave Rasa at home because it is a hot day. Tara and I leave for Woodland Hills and her appointment with Dr. Alice. It is over seventy degrees in Ventura, which it rarely is, and by the time we've gotten to Woodland Hills it is ninety-one. I'm happy with my decision to leave Rasa home in a cool house.

Tara is weighed. She has gained weight—probably a combination of no exercise, new higher protein food, and the extra food she has been getting. I make a mental note to adjust her diet accordingly. We are having a consultation today about the new cancer surgery and a treatment. Dr. Alice, always an attractive bundle of vibrant energy with sparkling eyes swirls in to the room. She opens the by now fat file and begins to look at Dr. Nicci's surgical notes. She finds the biopsy report.

She looks at Tara, "Has Tara aged since I last saw her?"

"Yes, she has," I answer hating to admit this.

"She has another soft tissue sarcoma, but it is different from the first one. This one is a grade one peripheral nerve sheath origin. It has dirty margins. Let me see the surgical site."

I show her the back of Tara's right hind leg.

"Above the hock."

"I won't amputate her leg. She would never get up again."

"How do you know that?"

"She won't get up with one of those post-surgical collars on her head."

"I've treated a couple of sight hounds that had a leg amputated and they never got up again."

"Catahoulas are sight and scent hounds. They live to chase and run."

"Oh, today is her regularly scheduled appointment. We'll do the scheduled treatment for her back, and start her on the new treatment for her leg today."

I move to the waiting room. Here we go: weekly trips, huge bills. I read a poster on the wall, "One in four dogs die of cancer. Fifty percent of all dogs over ten years of age will be affected by cancer."

At home I pull out the sheet describing soft tissue sarcomas that Dr. Alice originally handed me when Tara first saw her. I had marked what her first cancer was—neurofibrosarcoma: "Likely to recur and be locally invasive. Fibrosarcoma is a brutal killer. It may fool the best doctor because it recurs even after the best planned surgeries." I don't remember reading this. Tara's second tumor was a Schwannoma nerve sheath tumor: "Likely to recur and be locally invasive. It may behave insidiously. If the mass is on a leg, wide surgical margins are nearly impossible." I know this by now. I look at the description for Rasa's mast cell tumor: "The most fatal of all skin tumors in dogs."

Well, Rasa beat it. She is cured. But we waded through the full-on chemotherapy to get there. And I made a different decision for Tara because she isn't nine like Rasa was. She is twelve. This fight seems against all odds. I hate cancer. I hate that it killed my mother when she was fifty-seven. I hate that it may kill my sweet Tara.

I walk over to Tara's bed. I crouch down next to her. I hold my hands on her legs and I rub her body, which she loves. "Kundun, send her healing energy." I feel myself collapsing under this. I didn't give up on Kundun. I didn't give up on Genji. I didn't give up on Rasa. Rasa is cured. Genji is close to being back to his former fit self. Is Tara going to join Kundun? I have to think positively, stay in the present moment. I cannot give up on Tara—I owe her that for all of the wonderful years we've had, and because of her endless struggle with being abused, and how finally in spite of all her physical challenges during the past three and a half years, she has for the most part been free from the psychological trauma caused by her abusers.

46

Laura and I meet at the stable at nine-thirty in the morning. The day is sunny and clear with a light breeze blowing from the ocean.

"Genji, you look beautiful!"

Genji's mane now falls slightly past the top of his front leg. I keep it braided half the time which allows it to grow without tangling and hairs breaking trying to untangle it. I also use a conditioner.

"Yes, I think I finally have his feed and supplements absolutely right now. Let's walk over there so Genji can graze on what's left of the grass."

The rains have ended. The days are getting warmer, and the lush green valley is slowly turning golden. Genji is pulling on me so hard I can barely keep him next to me while we walk. As we near the large round pen, Laura asks, "Do you think we should turn him out?"

"Let's do that."

Genji rolls right next to us then wanders away sniffing the ground. "Does he run in a turn-out?"

"Yes, when it is cooler and when there are other horses being active." We leave the round pen and head to the grassy area surrounding the turn-out pens. It is cooler here. The round pen has a wood stake fence and no breeze blows there. Also the sandy surface reflects the heat.

"I want a turn-out with the bay horse with a white stripe on his face."

"Which horse is that?"

"I'm not sure, I'll have to look for it. Genji gets a turn-out next to that mare over there now."

"She only wants to talk about her lessons. I want to talk about nature."

"Maybe you can teach her about nature," Laura offers.

"She goes from her barn to the large covered arena and back. I've never seen her being ridden anywhere else," I explain.

"Do you ride with someone else on the trails?"

"No, other people's horses can't keep up with Genji and I hate to talk when I'm riding. I'm like Genji—I like to observe nature and be quiet."

"Do you tell anyone where you are going?"

"No. I used to leave a note on my kitchen counter at the ranch giving the date, time, and trail I left to hike on. Finally I realized it could be a week before someone found the note and I'd be dead, so I quit doing that. I quit talking to anyone here about riding on the trails because I got tired of the lectures about doing it. I used to ride alone for miles out in the desert in Nevada when I was twelve. It's become a life-long habit by now."

Laura looks at me assessing this information, "Well I guess maybe Genji would come back."

I change the subject. "Let's have Genji tell us a story."

"There was a fox with kits in her den. A hawk flew down to grab one of the young foxes. The mother fox bit the hawk on the wing and injured it, so it couldn't fly. Then the fox fed the hawk until it was healed and could fly away."

"Wow, what a story!" I exclaim.

"Genji," Laura asks, "is this a real story or did you make it up?"

"Another horse told this story."

"Did that happen here or somewhere else?"

Genji doesn't seem to know and it doesn't matter to him where it happened.

"There was a sick horse here that died," Genji adds. "I told it to go with the dog with the big ears. There are spirits of horses that have died here that are sad. I tell them all to go with the dog with the big ears."

"Where are these horses dying?" Laura wants to know.

"I don't know. That barn is suspect after I found the starving horse hidden in a dark stall. I saw a horse covered up with a tarp after it died over there between the barn and the gate to the road. It probably died from colic."

"Is the trainer still there?"

"No. He and his horses were here one week then they moved to a large equine facility in Burbank."

"Let's walk through it. First let's talk to Kundun."

"Ride your breath like the wind!" Kundun emphatically states. "You need to stretch!"

I quietly acknowledge that I do need to stretch. I have a beautiful place to do this in my home, but I am not stretching. "I will Kundun, I will. I promise." I need to stretch. I need to meditate. I struggle to fit everything I need to do into my days. I feel overwhelmed and tired.

Probably literally reading my mind, Laura says, "I am working with positive affirmations with my clients now. What I see is how people have negative thoughts like, my dog has cancer and she's going to die. The dog knows these thoughts and manifests them. So, say I thoughts. Genji, what should she say to you?"

"I have strong sturdy legs."

"You have sturdy strong legs," I affirm.

"Use the I."

"I have sturdy strong legs," I say.

"I have lots of friends," Genji adds.

"I have lots of friends," I state. "Okay I get it. I was a little slow there."

I wonder if the 'I have lots of friends' is for me or him. Genji says he has lots of friends, but since I moved here I haven't really made friends. I've tried but my years at the ranch have turned me into a hopeless recluse who would rather be with my dogs.

"Shall we head for that barn?"

The barn is empty. All of the stall doors are open. It is clean and waiting for horses to move in. Genji does not seem to want to be in this barn. He is charging toward the door at the other end. After we emerge into the sunlight I cannot seem to get Genji to calm down or slow down.

Laura takes the lead rope, "Genji, when you are walking with people you need to walk slower. People can't walk as fast as horses can." She continues her dialog with him in silence until we reach the tie-up rail. I take the lead rope and wrap it around the rail three times. I don't tie it because sometimes he becomes startled and spooked like a few days ago in the wind, and goes backward suddenly. If the rope isn't tied it unwinds and I can grab it. If it is tied he hits resistance which adds to the scariness and spookiness of whatever has happened. It works best to grab the rope and go back with him a step or two while reassuring him that he is okay.

"What are you thinking Genji?" Laura asks.

"It's interesting that people and animals walk differently."

"What did you feel in that barn?"

"There is a memory in there of horses that weren't loved."

"A memory can stay in a physical place?" I grasp at this concept. I realize that I have experienced this, but I did not know exactly how I was getting the information.

"Oh, let me show you what I found when I arrived this morning!" I go in the tack room and bring out a beautiful reddish brown hawk feather. "It was right there," and I point to the sandy ground on the other side of the tie-up rail.

"Is it a tail feather?"

"I think it's a wing feather," and I point at the different sides.

"That's really amazing that you found the hawk feather and Genji told the story about the hawk."

"Life is so magical."

At home I take Tara out on her leash to go potty. Back in the house I hold her and say, "My legs are strong and sturdy. My cancer is gone. I'm getting better every day. My body is healthy. I'm not confused. I'm happy."

47

omething has gone terribly wrong with Tara's second treatment on her leg. While I am out of town for only six days the treatment site has broken open, become infected, and smells. Her leg is swollen and hot to touch. It has been challenging for her caretaker to get her to eat, take her medications, and even to drink water. Her caretaker thought what was happening to her leg was a normal result of the cancer treatment. I called almost every day to check in on Tara. The caretaker never asked me one question, or made one comment about this situation. I am simply endlessly amazed at the seeming stupidity and negligence of people who are supposedly professional animal caretakers.

I take Tara to Buena the morning after I return home. She is given an injection of antibiotics and antibiotics to take home. "Two more days and she probably would have lost her leg," Dr. Jill states.

I clean it and apply hot compresses to her leg twice a day as instructed. It is challenging to get her to eat or take her supplements. I have to keep the soft collar-cone on to keep her from licking her wound. I take it off so she'll go outside, drink and eat, because she won't move with it on her head. All weekend I ponder this situation. I can't leave town to attend a nephew's college graduation without a medical emergency happening. I cannot subject Tara to the possibility of this happening again. I can't afford the endless vet bills that accompany the cancer treatments, and now the vet bills for the side effects of those treatments as well.

By Monday morning I have made my decision, and I call Dr. Alice's office, "Hello Dr. Alice, this is Louise, and I am calling to let you know that I am not going to continue Tara's treatments on her leg." I explain what has happened— the infection, the hole, the fever in her leg.

"When fever affects a tumor area it seems to cause regression and remission. This is called immunotherapy. Dr. Coley in the 1800's worked on this theory. This was before there were antibiotics. It is named Coley's toxins. So, the remaining cancer cells, because it was a dirty margin, could have been killed by the fever in her leg."

"You are making me feel better already."

"We call this a complication in her treatment, and I would not allow you to proceed with her treatment based on what happened."

So, now Tara is on the wings and a prayer cure. This is a prescription of faith, positive affirmations, and alternative remedies.

Meanwhile when Rasa comes home from being boarded at the same place, she keeps licking and licking her butt. I think her anal glands are bothering her, so when Tara goes in for a recheck, Rasa has her anal glands expressed. Meanwhile she has wet the bed three times in a week. I am prepared for this with potty pads, a towel and flannel sheet all on top of my bed. It has happened randomly so I always follow the procedure. After she wets the bed, I take her downstairs to go outside then leave her in the kitchen for the rest of the night. In the morning I notice little spots of blood where she has been laying. The following night I do extra damage control and add a potty pad beneath her hind end on top of the layers of potty pads, towel and flannel sheet. In the morning there is a little wet spot on the potty pad and a little blood.

Something is wrong.

Rasa goes back to Buena. She is diagnosed with an anal gland infection. Urine and blood samples are taken to cover every base. She is placed on antibiotics. It has become almost impossible to leave town. A second nephew's college graduation is in one week. I've shortened the trip to Denver to three days, and have a pet-sitter coming to the house. Tara will never go back to the kennel again.

Laura joins us at the house. "How are you feeling, Tara?"

"I was sick with cancer before, but feeling better now. I told Kelly that my leg was infected, but she said, 'No it isn't.' I thought I was going to lose my leg. If people spend the night at the house (kennel), I want them to pay attention to me. Lisa eats a lot of food."

"She brings food to the house?" I ask.

"No, she eats food in the cupboards."

"There's hardly any food here when I leave."

Tara continues, "The housekeeper has a clicking in her brain. The rhythm of her breathing is off."

Laura explains, "When dogs say someone has a clicking in their brain, they mean that the person is mentally unbalanced."

"Wow, they all say the same thing?"

"Yes."

"Her breathing is probably because she smokes. I think I need to let her go. She is strange and hasn't been here long. I saw Chatty this morning and I wonder what he might have said to Rasa and Tara. I haven't seen or heard the coyotes for a couple of months."

"When I saw Chatty, I told him I don't want to talk to him," Tara responds.

"Why?" Laura asks.

"Because I don't feel well and I don't want a coyote to know that. Kundun told me that he showed Chatty a new trail. He has babies. Why didn't I have babies?"

My mouth opens. I look at Tara, I look at Laura. "You had surgery so you couldn't have babies." I feel completely guilty explaining this. "When Wuli was six months old and she came into her first heat at the ranch, coyotes and foxes came right up to the house."

"Foxes too?"

"Yes, a red fox. You know, that's how they kill coyotes. The bounty hunters get a female dog in heat to lure in the coyotes then they shoot them. I don't think people understand how many squirrels, gophers, rabbits and rats they eat. They really keep the rodent population down."

"Rasa, Rasa come downstairs and join our conversation."

"Did you see Chatty?" Laura asks.

"We talked. He said he is eating avocados off the trees. He saw a bear do it. I want to go to the horse ranch." To Tara, "Cancer goes away if you say you don't have cancer even if you do."

"How do you feel, Rasa?"

"I'm fine. I want to go walking—my legs are getting stiff. We should have little bits of meat, listen to inspirational music."

"You have a list for me!"

"Genji is really feeling good!" Rasa adds.

"You're being quiet, Tara," Laura notices.

"I don't have anything else to say."

"Tell us a poem," I suggest.

"Sometimes I'm in pain then it goes away and I get tired, then hopefully I'll get better."

"Tara, you need to get on the bio-pad."

"I did, but it made me dizzy."

"Why should she get on the bio-pad?" Laura wonders.

"I think it helped cure Rasa's cancer."

"Shall we talk to Kundun?"

"I love you a lot Mom. Sometimes I really miss you and other times I'm filled with peace. You know how you have to try to be happy on earth? Well, it's the same here. I'm getting lots of energy now. I'm working on the land there and with you. Mom, the book is going to be big! A lot of people are going to want to read this. I'll watch over everything while you're gone. Have a good trip."

We listen to Laura's animal family positive affirmations on her Blackberry.

"Tara, what are your affirmations?"

"I calm myself by licking, yawning and looking away. I use the wind as breath. I feel sturdy and grounded. I am hopeful. I am a dreamer of good things. I smile inside. I get restful sleep."

"Rasa, what are yours?"

"I like the smile inside one. I like I forgive others."

"Why?" Laura asks.

"It is good for Tara. I find comfort in the moon."

"When it is full?" Laura interrupts.

"On a full moon I need a walk. I am beautiful. I breathe easily. I digest life easily. My mom trusts me. I'm well behaved at the horse farm. I'm predictable. I'm safe."

Laura leaves and I sit quietly to contemplate their beautiful affirmations. I realize how some of those affirmations deal with old painful situations and memories in their lives, as well as former behaviors. And is that not what we all strive toward; to heal our bodies, minds and spirits to become whole again? I too am hopeful and a dreamer of good things. I also smile inside and breathe easily. I try to forgive others. Their affirmations are my affirmations. To those I add a few promises. I'll plant flowers Rasa. I'll do it when I get back from my trip. I promise. I'll finish the porch with a gate Tara so you can enjoy going out there. I'll make the animal shrine. I promise. I'll start stretching and meditate more Kundun. I promise.

The day is long, it is nearing summer solstice. Purple Finches and Pacific-slope Flycatchers are nesting on porch ledges. A pair of Black Phoebes appears to be looking for a nesting site. A Great Blue Heron floats noiselessly down onto the hill above the house, takes several long deliberate strides and stands as still as a statue. Rasa and Tara think it is a Wild Turkey and want to charge out the door to chase it. That brings to mind our years of rides on high mountain trails; racing thunder storms home, sky growing darker, lightning flashing, thunder crashing behind us, plus miles and miles of hikes, turkey chases, rabbit hunts with Tara baying in the distance. I don't remember ever thinking that there would be anything else.

48

I t has been six weeks since Tara's leg became infected and the surgical site reopened. Dr. Nicci re-sutured it and put drainage tubes in it, which have now been removed. Tara has hot compresses with Epson Salts twice a day. A small area remains open and continues to drain.

When Laura arrives I have one question, "How does your leg feel, Tara?"

Tara looks at Laura, "You look different today, what are you eating?"

"Pizza," Laura answers.

"Don't eat pizza, it's not good for you. My leg feels fine. I don't know what all of the fuss is. I have a cranky feeling about going to the vet."

"What did the young coyote say?"

"How long have you lived here?"

I told him, "three years."

"Where is that funny looking dog?"

"He is in Heaven."

"That dog howled. Have you seen any rabbits?"

"I don't want to talk to you anymore."

Rasa and Tara don't howl now without Kundun. I always loved the sight and sound of the three dogs sitting in a group howling together whenever the coyotes began to howl. At the end of his physical life Kundun couldn't stretch his neck up to howl properly, so it sounded hoarse and shorter than his former deep, long coyote style howl.

Tara is very talkative today, "I had a dream about Kundun and he was being crushed by a half-elephant half-monster."

"Mom is going to a ball and I want to know what she is wearing," Rasa suddenly states.

"A ball? Oh, I'm going to a wedding next month."

"Wear a dress with a fluffy collar. I went to see that crazy Kelly. I was lonely without Tara there, but I had more room."

"Tara was boarded at the vet when I left for a few days in June," I explain to Laura.

"Let's talk to Kundun!"

"Anything special?" Laura asks.

"I've been missing him lately. I can feel him around, I don't know what he wants to communicate."

Kundun joins us, "Mom feels more joyful. Zuma has a string around his ankle. This grandchild is going to be different. Mom will get to spend more time with him. Genji needs to stretch his legs."

"I don't understand."

"He is showing me that you pull Genji's front legs out in front of him."

"Okay," I say skeptically.

Laura and I discuss the string around Zuma's ankle. We decide it is a spiritual thread.

Kundun continues, "Ganesha and I were fighting monsters that steal people's breath." I think of my asthma and how it steals my breath. Is that what he means? I like the concept of it portrayed as a monster.

"I tie up holes (that have been created) in auras from so much abuse that the soul is severed. I may look like a funny dog to you, but not in Heaven!"

"Tara, your eyes look softer. Are you calmer?" Laura comments.

"I'm giving her Rescue Remedy twice a day now."

"I'm starting to be more confident and courageous. It's easier to be brave than scared," Tara tells us.

"Do Rasa and Tara talk to Kundun?"

Rasa answers, "Yes, but he keeps changing shape and it's frustrating. I don't want to fight monsters in Heaven."

"What do you want to do?" Laura asks.

"I want to help hawks find nests, so that every hawk has a nest. I want to go to the big land with Kundun."

Tara answers, "I hang out with Kundun outside. We are falling in love all over again." We all spend time together outside. We talk about what direction the wind is blowing. We talk about crumbling."

"What is crumbling?" I want to know.

"When everyone does things over and over—repeating actions, thoughts, communications until there is a crumbling when you get fed up with what or how you are thinking," Tara explains.

Laura interjects, "She is giving me a visual of her flinching when someone comes near her."

Tara continues, "There is a pyramid in the mind's eye—the top is in Heaven. It crumbles down and you can't think at all. Then there is a light that goes up and a new way of thinking trickles down into the body, which gives a new awareness and a new way of being in your body, spirit and mind."

I sit shaking my head trying to not just grasp this concept, but that Tara knows this and communicates it so beautifully.

Tara isn't quite finished, "That baby that's coming is going to be wise, and you're going to teach him a lot!"

Our conversation ends all too soon leaving my head full of things to think about. I am especially touched by Tara's statement about falling in love with Kundun all over again. How did I not see their special feelings for each other all of those years?

49

Today at the stable it is overcast with a thin layer of clouds, so it seems cool beneath the pepper tree. We stay here for our conversation.

"What do you want to talk about?" Laura asks.

"I have a burning question. When I was out of town in May someone rode Genji. I want to find out what happened."

"How can you tell?"

"He won't let me put the bit in his mouth easily. The first time this happened was ten years ago. I've been taking the bridle home with me."

Genji and Laura's faces are very close. Genji plays with Laura's blouse with his top lip while they converse. "A young tall girl with straight blond hair got on me bareback. She didn't use a bridle, just a halter." Of course, I am horrified to even imagine a young person attempting to ride Genji. "I knew she was young and I needed to be careful. When she kicked me I put my head down and shook it." I am amazed. I do not know why Genji stood still so she could get on him and he is not a horse that needs kicking unless he is being stubborn about something that causes him anxiety.

"She got yelled at for taking the wrong horse. I was trying to tell Mom when it was happening."

"Is there another gray horse like Genji here?"

"Over in those corrals."

"Genji, why don't you let your mom put the bit in your mouth easily?"

"I wanted her to know someone else tried to ride me."

"Well, it worked," I acknowledge.

"I want Mom to bring a big can of supplements, so I can eat them out of the can."

"They are pre-measured for each day. I pour the contents of each individual packet into a zip-lock bag with a scoop of grain. Each morning he is fed one bag."

"I want more."

"You know Genji, how the other horses tell you that your eyes look so bright? Well, maybe they won't look so bright if you eat more."

"The other horses ask me if my mom will brush their tails. I tell them, 'no, she won't.'"

For me grooming Genji is a big part of our relationship. I always brush him including his mane and tail before we ride. After a ride I hose or sponge him off then apply hair conditioner to his mane and tail which I brush in. I spray an organic fly-spray with sun-screen on him and apply a hoof conditioner. I put aloe on any nicks or cuts. Finally he gets a clean fly mask and fly sheet. He looks very elegant when he goes back into his stall for carrots, apples and lunch—a single flake of grass hay waiting in his feeder.

"There are little spirits coming here."

Laura holds her hand about two feet off the ground, "How little? Like that?"

"Yes." Genji turns his head to look at the hillside past the end of his barn, and on the other side of the polo field/jumping arena. "They have sacred ceremonies up there."

"He looks at that hillside all of the time!" I exclaim.

"In the winter it is going to rain more than usual. There will be flooding. The little spirits are building walls to keep the water away from the horses. The fairies are coming back to earth now. They are coming to help with the chaos that is going to happen next year."

2011

"Wow, 2012. End of the Mayan calendar. This is really wild. Have you seen Kundun?"

"He is holding the portal open."

"What?"

Laura looks at me, "Kundun is holding the portal open—the doorway between the two realms—to let the little spirits and fairies through. She looks at Genji, "How come Kundun didn't tell us this?"

"Some things are supposed to be secrets. All of the people and animals and spirits will be able to understand each other."

"During my lifetime?" Laura asks.

"Yes, but it will be confusing at first with all of the voices, and there will be a lot of anger expressed. The ancestor spirits will return also."

Laura sees a horse being walked behind Genji's barn, "Let's go look at that horse."

The three of us walk around to the back of Genji's barn which is the side with the corrals. Every horse in the barn moves to the ends of the corrals where we are walking. They all watch Genji. The horse we are following is a handsome stud colt that belongs to the managers. He lives in the stall and corral at the end of the barn. We continue our walk around the end and back across the front of the barn to the tie-up rail. When I look back every horse is looking at Genji from the stall side.

"Look at that—he is the barn sage!"

50

The fog that has wrapped the valley in its cool cloak of mysteriousness every morning for the past two months is gone. Today the heat beats down on dried grasses and dusty earth pulling all of the energy out of everything that moves. Laura and I meet at the stable to talk to Genji.

"They didn't feed me today."

We survey the rest of the corrals in the barn. There is not one blade of hay in Genji's eating area. The other horses are nibbling on scattered pieces of hay. I see Mariano, one of the employees and call, "Mariano, did Genji get fed this morning?"

"Yes. "Yes."

"Que hora?"

"Seis y medio."

I know that Mariano looks after Genji, he works hard whether in the heat or rain. I put Genji's halter on and we all walk to the tie-up rail beneath the pepper tree. I take off his fly sheet and fly mask.

"Genji you look beautiful! Your eyes are so bright!"

I ask, "Why did we have such a difficult ride on Sunday? We rode on a different trail and all the way back Genji and I fought each other. He wanted to go fast and I wanted to go slow."

"The wind was angry."

"There was no wind in that canyon. The air was still and it was hot."

"There is anger here in the air. The owner is fighting with them."

"Do you mean the people who live in that little house?" and I point to it.

"Yes."

"So, the owner is fighting with the managers."

"He doesn't like anything they do."

"The managers have done nothing but make improvements here and the place looks beautiful now. I can't believe that."

"Maybe he should have a drink of vodka."

"Do you drink vodka?" Laura asks me.

"No, I drink sake."

"In a little shot glass?"

"Yes, is that what he is showing you? He saw that through the dogs' eyes and minds?"

Laura nods yes.

"I have no secrets! Zuma was born yesterday!"

Genji asks, "Are his eyes open?"

"Human babies are born with their eyes open," Laura explains.

"Does he see well?"

"Not yet, but he will," I answer.

"Is he going to ride a horse?" Genji wants to know.

"Definitely."

"When am I going to live with you?"

"I need to finish the book Genji. In a year we'll see what is happening."

"There is a chapter in the book called 'Genji,'" Genji remarks.

"Oh, Genji you have your own chapter," Laura exclaims.

"You will not believe this. There is a chapter with Genji written at the top, and it is sitting next to my keyboard on my desk ready to word process next!"

"Do you describe me?"

"Yes and how you looked when I first met you when you were young."

"Can I have a little horse?"

"I will get a little horse and it will be for Zuma to ride."

"I want a herd of horses."

"That would be fun wouldn't it," I laugh. While we converse Genji affectionately nibbles on the sleeve of my shirt with his top lip.

"Are the little spirits still here?" I ask.

Genji immediately turns his head to look toward the side of the hill beyond and above the jumping arena. He looks for a long time. "There are more spirits now. One of the spirits asked if he could ride me. I told him, 'yes'. The spirit said, 'Your mom will know if I ride you.'"

We all laugh.

"The spirits said for you not to worry or feel guilty about not coming to see me more than twice a week. They are watching after me now."

"Did you know that Tara and I fell down the stairs? I was trying to help her because she couldn't walk down. I put Rasa's harness on her and held the top of it, then Tara went too fast and we fell on the landing."

"I knew while it was happening. When you put anything around Tara's middle it brings back her bad memory of being kicked in the side."

"I thought she was kicked in the head."

"Maybe she was kicked twice," Laura offers.

I realize in this moment that yes, she was kicked at least twice and that bump on her rib that Dr. Jill said is an old injury is no doubt the result. I flash back in my mind to an incident at the barn on the ranch. Tara was in the tack room with the door closed because she hated the flies. I had a mare in the cross ties in the barn entrance while I was grooming her. Jake opened the tack room door and Tara ran out of the barn at full speed. This startled the horse and she jumped back so fast it broke one of the cross ties. Tara was terrified of Jake, but I didn't see it. I thought that he moved too fast around animals. I feel hopelessly stupid about not comprehending at all what this man did to my dog, and now eight years later still being confronted with it continuously. It's hard to forgive myself for this complete lapse of character judgment and awareness of Tara's behavior at the time.

Genji brings me back to the present moment, "Two girls were looking into my stall and said, 'Genji looks like a unicorn.'"

Laura adds, "He does look like a unicorn. I can see it—at night he grows his horn and his eyes turn into rainbows."

Genji gazes at Laura with deep, dark eyes, "Maybe I am a unicorn."

51

Rasa and Tara are on the front porch when Laura arrives. This is their very favorite place now that I have a wrought iron gate made for the opening by the driveway and a wrought iron continuation of the fence and railing across the front where I had gigantic rock stairs removed. A willow loveseat and two willow chairs with tropical floral patterned cushions are arranged in the center of the porch. A breeze seems to blow here continuously keeping the covered porch cool. Rasa and Tara each have a bed with a view into the oak grove next door and down into the area between the house and the street. There is a pile of rocks accumulated from the demolition of the stairs, which has now become a ground squirrel habitat. Beyond that and the low rock wall along the street glimpses of walkers, joggers, their dogs, and occasional horseback riders can be seen through the oak and eucalyptus foliage. I join Rasa and Tara here for lunch sometimes, or afternoon snacks, or what the locals call the "pink moment" at the end of the day when the hills magically turn a reddish pink color for a short time before sunset. The gate between the porch and their courtyard is always open now.

We settle in the kitchen and I begin, "We've had a lot of drama since you were last here. Rasa and Tara got into a huge fight in the kitchen right there," I point toward the space between their water bowl and the corner bed. "I don't know how it started, but Rasa was the aggressor. She had poor Tara spread-eagled on the floor on her stomach and was savagely biting her neck. I threw water on Rasa and got her out the door. The only reason Rasa didn't do any damage is because she is missing so many teeth. I had to towel dry the dogs, wipe up the floor and place the spray bottle on the counter, which is what I usually use for dog fights, but it was in the laundry room and actually they haven't had any fights for a long time.

"Since that fight Rasa began to stay outside all day every day which she was not doing before. Then Tara and I fell down the stairs when I was trying to help her get down them. I completely over-estimated how long of a walk she could take when Cassidy was here. I mean Cassidy's baby was due in ten days—how long of a hike was she going to take? I ended it because I was concerned about Tara's leg. The next morning Tara couldn't get down the stairs due to hind end mobility issues. Now I keep a gate across the bottom of the stairs when I'm not home.

Four days ago Tara had a seizure. I was here in the kitchen when it began, but I didn't see it. I heard her toenails clattering on the tile floor. By the time I rushed around the island, she was coming toward me, but she went by me toward the back door. I squatted down next to her and she started barking. That's when I noticed that her right eye was turned toward the outside of her eye socket, and that her back legs were not working right. I immediately thought, oh my god she's having a stroke! I helped her back into the kitchen, blocked off this area where the table and their beds are, then got her onto the corner bed. I was just leaving to go to LA to meet my grandson. Instead we went to the vet."

"I don't like situations like this," Laura emphatically states.

"Me either."

Laura then talks to Rasa for an extended period of time. Tara is in her bagel bed, and I am watching Laura and Rasa from my chair at the end of the table.

"I don't like Tara anymore. She gets too much attention. She smells bad."

"You're over-doing it Rasa. Tara isn't well. She had a seizure. You need to take care of her, not attack her," Laura instructs.

Tara speaks up, "I'm getting scared. I'm getting a metallic taste in my mouth. My head is making weird noises and my heart feels like it skips a beat. I've been scared all my life. I wake up sometimes and I don't know where I am. I still love my sister."

"How come she doesn't tell me these things?" Rasa asks.

"I ask her questions," Laura responds.

"Is Mom going to put her on an underwater machine? She needs to feel her legs move," Rasa suggests.

"Maybe we'll go to the Ventura River and wade across the Rice Canyon horse trail—it's deep enough that Tara almost has to swim."

"Tara's bed smells different," Rasa states.

"Like pee pee?" Laura asks.

"Like a different dog."

"She does smell strange. They had baths less than two weeks ago."

"I think Tara needs an adjustment from Steve. Maybe the fall down the stairs did something to her," Laura suggests. "Tara, you're going to go to Steve and he's going to adjust you. I'm sorry you got attacked."

"I don't remember most of it."

"Let's talk to Kundun," I interject.

"Maybe he can help us with this," Laura closes her eyes and makes contact with Kundun.

"I was with Rasa and Tara when you were gone. Tara's right side hurts from her eye down her neck and back to her tail. Zuma has a rattle."

"He is showing me an old looking metal rattle," Laura explains.

"My sister gave him a silver Navajo rattle. It's old. I don't know where it came from."

"Zuma is smart. He is already listening to everyone. He is talking to himself. He's strong and will walk early."

"Kundun is showing me a mirror, a big mirror?"

"Oh, Cassidy has the changing table on her bathroom counter and there is a mirror."

"Zuma knows it is his reflection," Kundun adds.

"I want to talk to Kundun," Rasa says as she pushes her head into Laura's lap.

"You can talk to Kundun."

"He's always so busy."

"I'm making sure the horses at the stable have clean water."

"Do they have automatic water?" Laura asks me.

"No, they have half-barrel plastic tubs that have to be emptied."

"Are they dirty?"

"It varies."

"You need moon energy to write your book. You need to twist for your lower back," Kundun instructs me.

Kundun is giving me lots of images today. He is saying that you need to clean off a table. Laura scans the dining table, but it is very organized today with piles of magazines, books and legal notepads.

"I think he means my desk and the top of the file cabinet-credenza next to my desk. They are fairly chaotic and messy with piles of paperwork that need filing.

"I love you and miss you Kundun."

"I love you and I'll always be with you and always take care of you. I can connect you to a higher realm if you want. What do you feel in your heart? Do you have a deep feeling that everything will be okay? You aren't supposed to struggle in this life."

"Some people are supposed to struggle in their lives," Laura comments.

Kundun signs off with, "The little spirits want you to read them a story."

Our time is up all too soon as always. After Laura leaves I reflect on our conversation. Tara breaks my heart. It was never possible to heal her wounds from the abuse, as hard as I tried. My guilt is impossible to quell because it all happened in our home where she should have been safe. How could I have so misread people? And Kundun, who could have ever imagined that rescuing a little scrawny puppy in a blizzard would evolve into having a special dog companion turned into protector angel, Ganesha's helper fighting monsters, removing obstacles, and offering guidance from Heaven? The little spirits want me to read them a story! I could be perceived as crazy, but what I do know is that I am privileged to be in a parallel reality and what exactly is reality? Reality is a perception and not necessarily a shared experience. Culture and religion are basically shared experiences, however there are always the fringe elements in culture and the mystics in religions who march to different drummers.

52

Rasa, Tara and I have our appointment with Cynthia today. It's a very hot day, ninety-nine degrees. We sit on the white wicker loveseat on her veranda while we wait for the door to open. Cynthia appears and we all go upstairs to her office.

"How is everybody?" No matter how hot it is or how warm her office may seem because the windows face west, Cynthia always looks crisp and cool.

"We're having problems since you last saw us. Tara had a seizure or maybe a small stroke because there seem to be permanent issues. Rasa has started two fights with her and their entire dynamic has changed. Rasa says she smells like a different dog. Tara does smell funny and I took her in for a bath even though she just had one two weeks prior. She can't stand up and turn in a circle anymore to change her position lying down. This creates problems with her ending up on top of me or Rasa at night. They sleep in the kitchen right now so that I can sleep. If I don't get my sleep then I'm cranky and don't get anything accomplished all day."

"Let's see what is going on here." Cynthia does some preliminary muscle testing on Tara. "She is missing one amino acid." Cynthia rummages around in her supplement cabinet which looks like a china cabinet. "This is the one."

She hands me two post-its with hieroglyphic arrangements of numbers to place in Rasa's and Tara's collars. She hands me a water-filled vial. When she turns on the tuning fork melody, I say, "Tara can't hear anything anymore."

"The vibrations will go into her body."

After testing with one stack of vial filled black boxes, Cynthia figures out what is happening with Tara, "She is releasing chemo-therapy toxins." By now Tara has moved over next to the desk. "I can smell her." Rasa is releasing old antibiotics, and you, my dear, are releasing old dental work and candida." Cynthia re-tests the amino acid, "After this work, Tara doesn't need to take this supplement." She holds up the white bottle and places it at the far end of her desk.

The dogs get their treats and we make an appointment for three weeks from today. We wade into the thick hot air and once in the car I blast us with the air-conditioning all the way home.

The following day we have our appointment with Steve. Rasa likes all of the attention she is getting from him. She thinks she is being rubbed and petted, however Steve is feeling her vertebrae. He adjusts her back below her shoulder blades, watches her walk and then does the same place a second time. Tara is afraid to go near Steve so we do a lot of maneuvering to get her to stand up, stand still, and keep her back straight. He feels her neck, "Her atlas and axis are out so I am adjusting them. This could have caused her seizure. Call me to let me know how they are doing in a few days."

By Monday Rasa and Tara seem more animated and able to move a little better. Tara begins to run down the hall with Rasa in the morning. This makes me smile. She becomes playful and silly before I feed them in the morning and again in the evening. She does a half jump-up with her shoulders and legs then dashes into the laundry room and back. She and Rasa play at the door while we are getting ready to go out just like the old days before every hike. I am so happy to see her act so energetic and young again.

After six nights in the kitchen I miss them sleeping with me and they happily join me in bed again. Tara comes with me to the bedroom and bathroom while I shower and dress after my morning tea in the kitchen like she used to. She also comes to my office while I am working which she hasn't done for a long time. The noise from the shredder bothers her so she would stay out in the hall stationed by the glass doors with a little Romeo and Juliet balcony overlooking the driveway and a partial view of the oak grove. Now she can't hear the shredder, so it no longer bothers her.

I decide to give Rasa and Tara a special treat and take them to the stable with me because it is foggy and cool. Genji is having a rest after his right shoulder seemed to bother him on our last ride. I am not going to ride so we will not be there long if the fog disappears and it becomes sunny. I give Genji a turnout, but all he does is roll. He absolutely loves to roll in the sand. I groom him and fix his supplement bags for the coming week. I take Rasa and Tara for a short walk where the ground is flat for maybe one hundred yards because I don't want Tara to overdo it.

Everything is okay until I watch Tara jump off the bed in the morning

WHY DO YOU NOT have Stairs for them?

and there is something slightly strange about how far out she jumps. Rasa and I go down the stairs, but I can tell that Tara can't get down. So, I encourage her and wait at the bottom. She keeps herself on her feet, but is out of control otherwise. I catch her at the bottom so she doesn't fall and they both go outside. I keep the stairway blocked with a wood folding gate, so she won't try to go upstairs.

Things decline rapidly. Tara begins to have trouble walking. Her head, legs and stomach begin to twitch and jerk not at the same time. She lies in her bed eyes staring straight ahead. Repeatedly during the day I sit on the floor next to her and stroke her body. By Monday Tara won't get up or walk. I call Laura who thankfully can stop by and help me get Tara in the car. We lift her into the back bed and all. I take her to Buena where they carry her in. She looks at me with frightened eyes.

After thoroughly checking her Dr. Jill explains, "It's neurological and it's her right side. The origin is in her neck or head. I suggest having her adjusted again." She flips through Tara's file. "She had those two sarcomas and they can be nasty." The expression on her face as she pronounces the word nasty says it all.

I make an appointment with Steve but I don't know how I'll get Tara in the car. I order a sling from a catalog wishing I'd done so weeks ago. Tara continues to eat well although a little less, drink water, pee and poop normally in spite of whatever else is going on. She gets out to the porch every day to enjoy being outdoors. I am so thankful that I finally accomplished doing this for her especially. But I never made her animal shrine and now I am filled with regret.

53

When you don't think one more thing can happen—it does. My car is rear-ended at a red light by a teenage driver. My bumper is damaged in a minor way, but his low small vehicle is impaled on my trailer hitch and tow hook, and is totaled. In the process of talking to the California Highway Patrol officer I have to explain why I have never gotten a California driver's license and I've lived here four years. Fortunately it isn't something you get a ticket for and ironically I had picked up the driver's handbook from the Motor Vehicle Department just within the past week.

After Tara's appointment with Dr. Jill and at the same time as my accident blood clots begin to appear in Tara's urine. I can only do one thing at a time. I decide that I will get my California driver's license first. I do that and make an appointment with Dr. Nicci for Tara. During this time I squeeze an appointment with Laura into the schedule because things seem to be spinning out of control for Tara.

"Is my sister going to die?" Rasa asks. "I look at her and I see death—like an organ popped."

"My whole body hurts. It hurts to pee," Tara tells us.

"I see death and around her body a darkness. I saw it with Kundun."

"My body feels sore and stiff when I move and my abdomen cramps."

"I want to take a walk. I need to get away from this. I want to go to the beach and look at a whale. I know we have a horse and he wants to move here. If Tara dies I'm the only dog in the house—what will I do with all of this room? Tara's going to Heaven soon. Tell her there's no fear in Heaven," Rasa blurts out.

"Tara, what are you thinking about this?" I ask.

"Sometimes I feel like I'm dying."

"You need to call the angels—she is dying!"

"Rasa never talks to me like this," Laura comments.

Rasa responds, "I didn't used to like you. I thought you were an all-knowing brat."

Laura laughs heartily at Rasa's comment. "Let's talk to Kundun about this."

"Tara doesn't feel well and there is a bed with a pillow here where she can rest."

"Does your bed have white sheets?" Laura asks.

"Yes, but not right now. The last change they were white."

"The bed Kundun is showing me has white sheets."

"Does Kundun mean that she goes there to rest then comes back?" I wonder.

"Her body is sick—she won't make it back."

Tara adds, "Sometimes I see all white and I get lost. I don't know where I am."

Laura tells her, "You have to let your mom know when you are ready—when you've had enough."

"If I feel like this much longer I'll be ready."

Laura asks me, "Has she had any more seizures since that one?"

"I haven't seen any, but that doesn't mean there haven't been any."

"They are inside her, not visible outside," Kundun explains.

"What do you want to say to your mom?" Laura asks Tara.

"I love you and I'm sorry I can't cuddle with you because it's painful to breathe."

"The bed is empty without you Tara. Even with Rasa there it is empty. I miss sleeping and snuggling with you. I love you and I'll always remember all of our hikes, and walks, and rides."

"I always remember them. Will I remember in Heaven?"

"Yes," I tell her.

"Are there men in Heaven? Will they hurt me?"

"No, they all went somewhere else," I assure her.

"There are angel-men," Laura explains.

"Can angel-men take away the fear instantly? I'm sad that I don't feel well. I wanted to take more walks. Is it bad to die?"

"No, it's beautiful. Just remember to go up through all of the levels fast," Laura responds.

"If she dies I'll take care of her," Kundun assures us.

"Are you going to get another dog?" Tara asks looking at me with deep, worried eyes.

"No."

"Not ever?" Laura questions in surprise.

"Probably not."

I don't explain to Laura or Tara that I don't want to die and leave a dog behind for someone else to care for, or that I'd like to stop having a dilemma about kennels and dog sitters—that I'd like to set the alarm, lock the door, and leave without the worry, the fear and the guilt, or that I never, ever want to experience the extreme heartbreak of having a dog of mine abused at home by someone working for me. It is very simply the most evil thing I have ever encountered in my life. On the other hand I cannot imagine life without a dog.

54

Fall equinox arrives with a shred of dawn at six. I hurry to the kitchen guided by night-lights in the hall. Rasa goes outside while I clean up Tara's potty pad. There is no blood clot. Tara is in her bed, then gets up to drink water and go outside. I follow her in the semi-darkness but it is too dark to see. We return to the kitchen. I make my tea and feed Rasa and Tara their meal. From the laundry room window I see the sky fill with rose and coral as the sun rouses itself.

When it is light enough I go outside to look for a blood-clot—none. As I walk through the wrought iron gates between the porch and the courtyard I see a brilliant, perfect rainbow toward the west above the hill behind the house. There are almost never rainbows here. A breeze fills the wind chimes with music, raindrops sprinkle, and it is the most magical moment. "Oh Tara, this is for you!" I wipe tears from my eyes. It is a sign from the Divine. In my heart I feel that either everything is going to be better for Tara, or Heaven is ready for her to arrive. While I shower and dress thunder booms and crashes. There is never thunder here. I don't think Tara can hear it now, but I hurry to be with her. I miss the thunder and rainbows in New Mexico.

On Saturday Dr. Nicci diagnoses Tara with a urinary tract infection and prescribes Cipro. After the first pill Tara has a considerable improvement. By afternoon she is a different dog acting playful. She goes to Steve for an adjustment Monday. He works on her while she stands on the tailgate of my SUV. She goes to Cynthia for sound balancing Tuesday. As with Kundun, Cynthia has moved her office to her living room. It is light-filled with lace curtains cascading across windows and Victorian furniture arranged for the view and conversation.

"She is detoxing chemo out of her spine now."

On Wednesday Dr. Liz Fernandez, the acupuncture vet, arrives at the house to treat Tara. Petite and dynamic she unloads her medical bag on wheels and rolls it into the kitchen. She takes very detailed notes about Tara's recent medical history then gives her a physical exam.

"What is your goal for her?"

"To give her some mobility and pain management."

We pull the corner dog bed out of the corner and into the center of the kitchen area where the dining table is. First Dr. Liz uses a hand-held battery-run low energy laser which she holds above Tara's vertebrae and moves it up and down her back. She hands a smaller one to me to use over her head between her ears. "This will stimulate her nerves."

Then Dr. Liz pulls out her needles and begins to insert them along Tara's spine, a couple in the top of her head, and more in her right hind and right front legs. She sets her timer for twenty minutes and we attempt to keep Tara quiet by petting her and feeding her an endless stream of her kibble. After the twenty minutes is finally ended she shows me a few techniques to stimulate the nerves in her back and feet, "Do these twice a day and I'll see her in two weeks. Take her on walks. She needs to walk."

At first after the treatment, Tara can hardly move and I panic. By the following morning Tara is managing the steps down into the courtyard and acting more animated. By dinnertime she is being playful and silly. It's a miracle. I move my hand along her spine pulling up skin and muscle with the tips of my fingers. I do this repeatedly and am fairly surprised when I realize that it is generating heat in her back and in my hand. I place my now warm hand on top of her head and massage it because this heat that has been generated is chi energy. I do this several times a day.

By the following day Tara walks much better, even runs for a short distance simply for the joy of it. She joins Rasa and me for the walk to the side of the garage at night, and is very disappointed that she is not coming upstairs to bed with us. As if life is normal again Tara has a bath and we take a short walk.

Ten days later a coyote trots across the top of the property. I let Tara out the door—she could use a little excitement in her life right now. Tara runs straight up the hill to the fence. I don't think her feet touch the ground. She flies each leg and foot looking like nothing is wrong. I hold my breath. She barks at the coyote that has now ducked into the brush. She makes her way back down stumbling a little. My heart smiles for my hound.

I think of the rainbow, the Divine giving me the courage to not give up and the hope that whatever happens—it's okay—just ride the wave wherever it's going.

55

September slips quietly into October. Days shorten and shadows lengthen as the sun sinks toward the south. The coastal mountains and valleys remain hot as the burning Mojave Desert air expands west. Along the coast there is a cool whisper of winter on its way promising to bring relief to parched meadows where Turkey Vultures cruise on thermals in their endless search for inert life forms.

Laura arrives at the house for our conversation, "Tara how are you feeling?"

"The last time you were here, I thought I was going to die. Now I'm going to live until snow."

"It doesn't snow here."

"She means winter," Rasa explains.

"I want real meat—I'm hungry," Tara adds. "My back hurts and I'm thirsty all the time."

"The baby is really smart. He kept saying dog, dog, dog and wanted to pet me," Rasa exclaims. "He cries and says my hip hurts—his left hip and lower back. He said, 'I want to ride a horse. I am an engineer.' He is smarter than his mom and dad together. I want chicken treats. Is Mom going to brush my teeth again?"

"My whole body feels tight. I want acupuncture on my elbow," Tara says.

"Genji is angry at the ground—it's changed," Rasa tells me.

"One of his shoes got bent somehow. Tano is going to fix it. Are you okay in the kitchen, Tara?" I ask.

"The night is long. I wake up and miss you. I'm okay though."

"I wake up and miss you too."

"I saw Kundun's coyote friend, Chatty, and he wants a bucket of water," Rasa adds.

"The last time I did that there were hundreds of ants, but I'll try it again."

"The baby is going to make everyone tired. I'm having trouble getting in the car," Rasa confesses.

"Also up and down the stairs and on and off the bed," I add.

"My body feels really good—I just can't jump as high. There is a sound in my ear every few days then it goes away."

To Laura I say, "She is losing her hearing. I have to go outside to the porch and call her name or she doesn't hear me."

"A spirit follows you around and tells you to write. When you write you're fine. When you don't write steam comes out of your head," Rasa says.

At first I am baffled, then laugh. "Chicken livers exploded in the microwave. What a mess!"

"The needles go whoosh. Tara goes from black to rainbow with acupuncture. Mom keeps saying we are old dogs. I want you to stop saying that."

"I call myself old too. Do you want me to call you puppies?" I tease.

"Say mature."

"Let's talk to Kundun," I suggest.

Kundun joins us, "I am not working so much. I am resting now with you. I want you to focus your eyes."

"Does he mean you aren't in your body?" Laura asks me.

"I think he is referring to how I stumbled into the wrought iron gate when I was pulling the hose to the porch to spray off Tara's pee. The hose scared Tara and in the process of trying to avoid her I knocked a chunk of skin off my arm."

Kundun continues, "I'm hoping to stream energy and I want to be with my family. Genji is safe and happy at his stable. The dust from the equipment is making his eyes runny. He isn't upset at the horse that bit him. Cassidy is happy to have you as her mother."

On the weekend I push the futon mattress against the wall of the small room next to the kitchen and make it with the same soft blue chambray sheets and red plaid duvet cover that I had in my tipi in New Mexico. I bring the pillows down from my bedroom and place the dog blanket on the wall side of the bed plus a towel for padding against the wall for Tara. We all settle in for the night. The last time I slept on this futon was in my tipi at the ranch with Rasa and Tara years ago. I thought it was comfortable, cozy and wonderful. Maybe that was due to being outdoors in the mountain air with a campfire and the dazzle of the Milky Way visible through the open top flaps.

"Let's pretend we're in the tipi tonight!" Maybe I sleep two hours. Tara snuggles up to me ecstatic to be sleeping with me again. Rasa keeps walking off the futon and back on—off and on. She finally settles down. The night finally ends. My attempt to sleep with Tara isn't as successful as I had hoped and I am disappointed. Not one to give up easily I find a super-padded bed pad in a catalog and order it. Overflow houseguests will also probably appreciate it.

The nifty new harness for Tara arrives. It is black and gray with a padded strap around her back and chest and a second one around her back and belly. There is a V-shape piece on the front of her chest below her neck to hold it in place and a sturdy handle in the middle of her back. At first she is reluctant to walk, however we are headed for the car and she loves to go with me. Getting in I still have to grab her rear end and give it a boost, but getting out it is like she is on a parachute. All four feet touch down at the same time. Once she realizes that the harness helps her she is eager to walk while wearing it. Hooray we are mobile!

56

"Hello Genji, how are you? You look beautiful!" Laura, Genji and I walk past the small covered arena and the large round turn-out pen. On the far side of the round pen grass and other plants have begun to grow after our first rain two weeks ago. Genji begins to graze. "What do you want to talk about?" Laura asks.

"What do the little spirits say?" I curiously inquire.

Genji doesn't answer this he has something else on his mind. "The young girl has a job somewhere else. She is saving money so she can move away from here. She isn't happy."

Kimberly has in fact become a mystery. She is never around anymore and boarders have speculated that she is working somewhere else. Meanwhile, another young lady who rarely smiles or says hello takes each of the managers' horses out of its corral, grooms it and puts it back one after another. Sometimes a horse is saddled and unsaddled without being ridden.

"The little spirits like it here," Genji reports.

"Sunday Genji and I were standing here while he dried off from a sponge bath after our ride up to the power line tower. I looked up at that road that goes straight up the mountain." I point past the barns and at the mid-section of the steep hillside. "Something that didn't fit in caught my eye. I stared and stared at a shape that appeared to be a reddish brown animal sitting near the side of that road. Too large and too reddish for a coyote. Didn't move. It had to be a mountain lion. I watched a mountain lion on my ranch and a Bengal tiger in India—they don't move, not even an ear. My eyes ached from staring at a shape I could not see clearly. I looked away, moved Genji a few steps, looked back—gone! They know you are looking at them."

"The mountain lion walks through here at night," Genji tells us.

"What do you do?" Laura asks.

"I go in my stall and close my eyes."

"Tell us a story Genji."

"There is a little pony here and the pony wanted to be a big horse that could jump. He was very unhappy with his short legs and not being a jumper. Then one day a young girl rode him and jumped him. The pony said, 'See, if you dream about something it will happen.'"

"Oh Genji what a great story!" I respond.

"Where is the pony?" Laura asks.

"I don't know. I haven't seen a little pony here," I answer. "Tara is off."

"What do you mean?"

"She isn't eating well. I'm worried about her."

"Tara will get better. The damp, foggy weather made her feel bad," Genji assures me. "The baby has pain deep in his ears. That's why he is so fussy. Are you at the place in the book where Kundun meets the elephant man?"

"Not yet. I'm at the place where Dr. Sherry treats you. After that is when Kundun gets very sick."

"Dr. Sherry knows how to treat animals. She told me that when horses are born vertebrae in their necks can be dislocated."

Two beautiful mares, a reddish Thoroughbred, and a black half-Arab half Friesian, are led past us from the turn-out pens back to their stalls in the large barn. "They won't talk to me because I don't get turn-outs anymore. They say I don't know how to talk."

"If they told you that then they are talking to you," Laura states. "Why isn't Genji getting turn-outs anymore?"

"His behavior changed. He wouldn't walk up to me anymore."

"I played so much in the turn-outs that I was too tired to go riding."

"I don't believe that. I think he was being handled improperly. The minute I stopped the turn-outs he was fine again."

"My bit is hurting my mouth."

"Oh dear and you've had the same bit for thirteen years."

"I want something gentler on my mouth. I want a new brow band."

"He is showing me a multi-colored woven brow band."

"I don't know where to find one like that."

Our session ends and we walk back to Genji's barn. "Didn't Genji tell us that there would be ponies here?"

"Yes, and lots of young people, which there are. They take lessons from Shelley."

After Genji is back in his stall I prepare his week's bags of supplements. I rummage through my tack box and much to my surprise I find a new Mylar bit that I had bought years ago but never used and had forgotten about. I put the bit and bridle in my car, sweep the tack room and am just turning to leave when Shelley calls to me.

"Come see what I teach my students."

I walk over to the large round pen where a ten year old girl is standing in the center with a whip while an Arab gelding bucks and gallops wildly around her in circles.

"When a new horse is introduced to the herd, what do the other horses all do? They chase it until it figures out its place in the herd hierarchy. She is chasing it with the whip," Shelley says to me. Then she focuses on her student, "Okay now he is going to be submissive toward you. See, he stopped and is turned toward you. Drop the whip!" The horse walks toward the girl.

"Is he licking his lips? Yes, see now he is licking his lips. Rub him on the neck. Now walk over here." The horse walks right behind her. "Now run!" The horse trots behind her as she runs up to the gate where we are standing. Shelley has filmed the entire sequence on her phone. "I put this to music as a video and it makes you cry when you watch it. It makes me cry."

As I drive out I see a young girl put a pinto pony in a corral. That must be the pony in Genji's story. It isn't little like a Shetland pony but it is smaller than Genji. I think about the girl in the round pen and wish I would have had a teacher like Shelley. I learned to take care of a horse and ride without the benefit of a teacher or lessons until I got my first gaited horse when I was nineteen.

57

I have interviewed a new pet sitter because Lisa is busy with her graduate school and can no longer take care of Rasa and Tara. Laura arrives for our last session before she takes a two month leave to work on a book she is writing.

"Brandy, who you met yesterday, is coming to stay while Mom leaves for two weeks."

"Are you going to give her a description so she doesn't get us confused?" Rasa wonders.

"Is she going to touch me?" Tara asks.

"She is going to massage you. She is certified in dog massage," I assure Tara.

"What if she hurts me?" Tara wants to know.

"You need to let her know if she hurts you, so you can growl at her," Laura instructs.

"Is she going to give us our supplements?"

"Tara is showing me an orange looking gel-cap and wants to know where that is."

"I wonder if she means the Hepato which I quit giving her when she got sick and wouldn't take her pills anymore. It's for her liver. I'll try sprinkling it on her food like I do a couple of other supplements."

"Yes, she'll give you your supplements," Laura says.

"Are you going to talk to us every day?" Tara asks me.

"Yes, at night." Before I ever moved to California or met Laura, when I traveled I would visualize each dog and try as hard as I could to give them a visual expression of my love. I never knew if I had been successful but I would drift into sleep feeling close to them.

"Tell her I want walks!" Rasa emphatically states, "Where are you going?"

"I'm going to Hawaii to the beach."

"I've never been to Hawaii—I'd like to go there."

"It's a tough trip for dogs. You have to fly in an airplane in a crate. It's dark and it takes a long time. We'll drive to a hotel on the beach. I promise."

I think of how I thought the dogs and I would take driving trips to different places after we moved to California. We'd explore and take walks, stay in hotels that allow dogs. All's I've done for three years is help one dog after another through one medical crisis after the next. There was no extra money to go anywhere—it all paid the vet bills.

"I want my picture in the book—a full page and I'll have wisdom with it. This is the wisdom: 'Dogs know people's minds better than people know dogs' minds, so they need to listen when they are sleeping or after they eat.'"

"Okay Rasa, I'll do that. Thank you for your wisdom."

"When you are sleeping I go into your mind between dreams and tell you, 'Let's take a walk!' You need to eat more vegetables—the kind that are squishy."

"She is showing me something like squash."

"You are too stressed," Rasa adds.

"I am stressed. The car is in the shop being repaired after I was rear-ended at the stop light. I hate the rental car. The washer has been broken now for three weeks and I have to keep going to the Laundromat. I've spent so much money trying to get it repaired that I may as well have bought a new one."

"Let's check in with Kundun."

"Alan misses you. When you get stressed you can think of me. You have a rock the color I am and you can rub it."

"Do you have rocks?" Laura asks me.

"I do. I have lots of rocks. I'll have to look—I don't remember a brindle color rock."

Kundun continues, "Tara wants to go upstairs. I don't think she should. Tara can't eat too much, it hurts her stomach. You are going to meet a nice man and he will be talkative."

Startled, I look up at Laura and laugh "Where am I going to meet anyone—I'm completely anti-social."

"You have a sun in your heart and you should let it explode. Alan wants to meet his cousin. He is sad that he isn't coming for Christmas."

"I am too. How is Bhakti?"

"Bhakti is in a place in Heaven with his family—where they're good—where it is the best of everybody."

I look at Laura, "I don't understand. Is he with a different family in Heaven?"

"It's his family, and the way dogs explain this to me is that in Heaven there is a mirror of this realm which isn't separate. The higher self is there, and Bhakti is with the higher selves of his family."

I quietly reflect on this. "Are you happy, Bhakti?"

"I feel happy and I care about myself here."

"I love you, Bhakti. We all miss you."

"Thank you. You helped me keep living and taught me what real love is. I'm working on letting go of sadness."

November brings cooler weather with rain. Thanksgiving is a noisy family filled weekend with Zuma now three months old, Cassidy and Alex, plus my brother, his girlfriend and my nephew. Tara holds court in her bagel bed in the kitchen corner. I rearrange the table and chairs to accommodate her. Not a very social dog, she seems to accept and enjoy the presence of family and is particularly curious about Zuma. When he is in my lap Tara takes a few steps out of her bed and sniffs the top of his head. Of course, Rasa and Tara always love the turkey treats that come with the arrival of holidays and family.

58

I leave for Hawaii with much apprehension about leaving Tara in the house alone with a new pet sitter to care for her and having planned a two week trip, which I cannot change now. Rasa stays with Kelly because I want no opportunity for a dog fight to arise under any circumstance at this point. I call Brandy every day to check on Tara. As the time goes by Tara begins to eat more, walk up the hill in the yard regularly, and act playful. Brandy spends a lot of time with her and falls completely in love with her. During this time Brandy finds out that her mother has terminal cancer. She alternates between being at the hospital in Ventura with her mother and taking refuge at the house with Tara. I send Tara and Rasa messages of love every morning early. I chant our positive affirmations to them.

I become apprehensive about being gone so long, but when I try to change my hotel reservations and airline ticket I discover that I will have to pay for the room anyway and the airline ticket magically becomes one way so that I will have to pay the full fare again. This is when I discover that I can't count, and not only can I not leave early—I have made my trip plans for fifteen days not fourteen. I call Brandy to explain my math problem and try my best to enjoy family, Christmas shopping, and being in such a beautiful place while I worry about my beloved Tara.

When I arrive home in the morning Tara doesn't know who I am immediately. She looks at me questioningly as she gets out of her bed. I squat by my chair at the table in the kitchen and she flops on her side on the rug there and makes little joyful grunts and moans of happiness. I rub her tummy and we hug and kiss. I see that she has lost weight, but her eyes are bright. We go outside together. I leave her on the porch while I unpack and do laundry. I pick up Rasa in the afternoon. She barks and barks and runs to the gate at the kennel to greet me. I pack her gear in the car and off we go. It's good to be home with my girls.

First, Tara stops eating her food. I decide to change her diet and get some canned food for her to try. Next, very loose stools appear. I immediately put her on Bio-sponge and exchange the cans for something less rich. She pees and poops in multiple places in the kitchen. I leave Rasa on the bed asleep and head downstairs to clean up after Tara. Tara eats more and seems to digest her food better. Finally we have two nights of no mess and dry potty pads. She is enjoying hours on the front porch every day.

Five days after being home I take Rasa and Tara to the stable with me. After I give Genji a turn-out, groom him and take him back to his stall for apples and carrots, I walk Rasa and Tara across the grass to his stall door to say hello. Then we take a small walk because Tara seems frail. The following day Tara spends all day on the porch happy to be outside, and as always, looking for those squirrels in the rock pile.

Seven days after getting back, a coyote appears on the hill above the dog yard. There is a barking commotion in the kitchen. I let them out and they charge up the hill. Tara trots along the fence barking. The coyote heads up the hill and disappears into the brush. Rasa comes back to the door, but Tara stays at her post awhile longer. I watch her and think, "Oh wonderful, she's getting stronger and feels much better." However, she leaves half her morning meal and again half her dinner.

I massage her at bedtime and recite her positive affirmations, "I am beautiful. I smile inside. I am hopeful. I am a dreamer of good things. I forgive others. I am safe. I am loved. I am home." I always repeat the last three, "I am safe. I am loved. I am home." I adjust the downstairs furnace thermostat. I turn up the radiator-like space heater I have in the kitchen for her. I leave the light over the stove on low. I look back from the door, "Nighty-night sweetheart. I love you." I silently climb the stairs. Rasa waits for me at the top.

In the morning again there is no mess. The potty pads are dry. She stays in bed while I fix my tea and feed Rasa. After she eats Rasa goes outside. I look at the thermometer. It is forty degrees. I coax Tara into getting up to go outside. I'm not sure why but I turn away from the door rather than go out with her as usual. When I look out moments later Rasa is at the door, but Tara is next to the planter several feet away from the door her back legs wobbling, careening, collapsing.

"Oh my God!" I open the door to let Rasa in and help Tara get to the bed in the corner by the heater. I rush to get her harness hanging on a hook in the back hall—she's not going to be able to move without it. When I return to her side she has thrown up a little white residue of her pain pill from last night. This incident has scared her, but why wasn't that digested after twelve hours? I clean it up and try to get the harness on her. She growls while I am trying to get one of the straps around her belly. It must be painful.

I look at the clock—seven A.M. I sit at the table and try to drink my tea with the realization of what this means dropping over me like a heavy, dark, suffocating blanket. "Oh Tara." Tears well up and overflow moving slowly toward my chin.

Tara licks her mouth. She is thirsty. I wash the water bowl and fill it with clean filtered water. I carry it over to her, but she refuses to drink. I place it in its customary place six feet from her bed. I finish buckling up her harness and she struggles to get up. I grab the handle and help her get to the water bowl. She drinks and I get her back to and settled on her bed. Tara through all of her illnesses has always had a very clear and resolute understanding of where she eats and drinks, of what is normal.

The clock erratically crawls and speeds to eight A.M. I call Buena, "Hello, this is Louise. I'm going to lose it, so stay with me. I need to make an appointment to have T—Ta—I'm sorry—Tara eu—eu—thanized today." I try to get the words out between sobs.

"Dr. Nicci is available at 10:50 A.M. or 2:30 P.M."

"Oh, Dr. Nicci is there today? I don't know. This morning is too soon. I'll take the 2:30 and I want it done in the car. I don't want her to go in there again." I remember all too clearly how Tara did not like Kundun's euthanasia on the floor of the operating room, and neither did I. We've been driving around in the car for five years, so it's practically an extension of the house. I hang up and look over at Tara.

I walk over to her and sit on the floor. "Tara, it's time to go be with Kundun now. I'm sorry, I'm so sorry. You've been brave and valiant, courageous and strong. Oh Tara, I'll miss you for the rest of my life. I love you so much."

I shower and dress remembering how Tara would come upstairs to join me. She would peek her head around the open air shower door to see if that is where I was because she couldn't hear the water then she would lie on the bathroom rug in the morning sun. I have missed this for the last four months, as well as her joining me in my office while I work, and of course sleeping with me every night cuddling up next to me.

Back in the kitchen I help Tara move to her bagel bed. I believe in having ordinary last days. There is a mysterious comfort in going through the motions of what it is we do. So, I leave Tara in her bed in the kitchen and go to my office to take care of some work. I am thankful for having my Christmas gifts all wrapped by now. I did that at the kitchen table with Christmas music on the stereo, Rasa and Tara watching me from their beds. I didn't put the little fake tree on the kitchen counter yet, and because I am going to Cassidy's in LA for Christmas I'm not having a real Christmas tree this year.

I help Tara out of her bed and out the door. We manage the steps and through the gate to the front porch. She walks with her front legs and I hold the rest of her up with the harness. I adjust the straps yet again she has lost so much weight by now. I get her situated in her bed and go back inside. I decide to check on her one more time and somehow she has managed to walk across the porch! I help her lie on the other bed with a much better view of the rock pile plus some warm winter sun on solstice.

We drive to Ventura. "It's a beautiful day Tara. It's sunny. The ocean is calm. The Channel Islands are wrapped in fog and mist." Rasa lies next to Tara in the back. I park behind Buena in the shade of a large eucalyptus tree.

In the clinic I am numb. "I'm here with Tara. The car is in the back. I want her to have a private cre—cre..." Unable to even say the word, I become silent. I sign the paperwork and pay Tara's last expense at the vet.

I open the top half of the back of my Landcruiser and open the door behind the driver's seat. I sit there and pull Tara's head onto my thigh. An ocean breeze blows into the car. I try to surrender myself to this moment as painful as it is. "You'll be with Kundun again Tara. You'll be able to hear and run—be free of the pain. I'll always miss you Tara. I'll have a hole in my heart when you are gone. Thank you for all of the years, the wonderful years of life with Miss Tara. Dolly Girl. Miss Patuti. The hikes, the rides, the walks, the trips. I never made the animal shrine for you. I'll make it and it will be Tara's animal shrine. Oh Tara."

With my heart aching as if I am losing my own child, and words no longer able to manifest in my mind or mouth, I begin to rub her lightly and say our positive affirmations, "I am beautiful. I smile inside. I am hopeful. I am a dreamer of good things. I use the wind as breath. I forgive others. I am safe. I am loved. I am home."

That night I am in bed and cannot sleep for what seems like hours although I am comforted by Rasa next to me. "Tara I miss you so much. I love you. This is so hard." Magically Tara sends me the most amazing image. It is a view of a beach looking down the shore with the ocean on the right and the sand in little wavy dunes extending along the ocean in front of me. There is a winding trail of sparkling red lights on the sand and next to it is a winding trail of sparkling smaller green lights. I immediately realize that Tara has sent an exquisite Christmas card symbolizing the two of us walking on Santa Claus Beach in Carpinteria.

59

"After Kundun's death, he said, 'Be happy. Take care of Mom.' That's what we have to do Rasa. Be happy, and you need to take care of me." I also need to care for myself. I lost ten pounds worrying about and caring for Tara after her seizure. I find the stone Kundun told me to hold in my hand when I am feeling stress, although by now it is more of a feeling of overwhelming sadness. It is actually a large, oblong ivory shaman bead that I bought from a merchant of illegal items in Burma. A sign posted on his table in the market said, "No Photos." I didn't realize it was ivory when I bought it. It has been on my bedroom altar for years. I pick it up and hold it next to my heart. Somehow Kundun has blessed it to ease my suffering. It feels smooth to touch, is kind of a brindle color, and seems very old. It has the power of elephant energy within it.

Rasa and I go through our days. I give her a lot of love and attention. She spent her entire life wanting to be an only dog, however, I can plainly see that being the only dog does not make her happy. She grieves the loss of Tara so much I am concerned about her well-being. I reflect on the irony of the fact that Rasa was the only dog I planned to have. The breeder talked me into taking Tara as well since she would be the only puppy left. Then Kundun came into our lives and quite honestly I cannot imagine my life without the company of these two special beings in dog form, and I'm certain neither can Rasa.

Tara manifests her love for me in mystical ways. At Suzanne's I order a grilled salmon steak salad and request all romaine lettuce. As I am eating I find a tiny heart shaped piece of dark green—I have no idea what, but I know one thing for certain—it is from Tara. I reflect on the date today, the third of January. Twelve years ago today I rescued Kundun and he became an integral part of our family. I find it hard to believe it has been twelve years. He lived his life and is gone now, or at least from this realm.

Laura arrives for our conversation. Rasa is on the porch, so we walk out the kitchen door and around to the porch where Rasa is still barking at Laura's car parked in the driveway. Rasa is excited, "I see Tara a lot and her head isn't injured anymore." Back in the kitchen Rasa adds, "When Tara died I saw her spirit leave and it went right through me. When I see her sometimes she and Kundun are playing tug-of-war. She doesn't have that look on her face."

"What look?" Laura asks.

"Of fear. There is a different group of people at the stable and they all think I am beautiful. I want new snacks that are different and chewy. I want a new toy. All of the old toys smell like Tara."

I ask, "Are you okay now Rasa with Tara gone and being the only dog?"

"There are lots of empty places now where Tara used to lie, but Kundun and Tara come to visit me and then I feel better. You are such a great mom and the way you took care of Kundun and Tara when they died—I know I'm not afraid to die. I know I'll be safe. Tara loves you. You are too hard on yourself."

"I am. I'll try to stop doing that."

"Let's talk to Tara," Laura enthusiastically offers. Laura talks to Tara for a long time. She looks like she is going to cry.

"After I died I walked slowly in a bright, light space like fog. I walked up a slight incline—not a hill. Then I saw Kundun and he came running up to me. We walked together slowly with Kundun on my left. I saw Mom up in front of me and I went to her."

I look at Laura with a question on my face.

"Your higher self."

"She told me everything she loved about me and my life with her."

Laura explains what she sees, "Tara is absorbing peace and is in a meditative state. She isn't where Kundun is, but they interact and come together. Tara settles down with you. You hold her and she curls up with you like spooning."

Kundun adds, "Tara will transform and move out of that place, but never go where I am because it's a busy, busy place.

"Like a pinball machine," Laura exclaims.

"I love you Tara. I miss you so much."

Laura responds for Tara, "Your love for her is like blood pumping through her, but she doesn't have or need blood there, so it's like an essence, an energy. She has all of her memory from her past. She is filled with love and is joyful. She misses her routine at home. She has a routine there, but it is a different routine."

"I manifest in dog form, but in Heaven I feel like a wise old man. I am a contained energy that is like electricity with flashing lights and currents going through it. I can make things move faster—speed up a process. When I was walking with Tara many different beings were giving me offerings of energy, which I gave to Tara."

Laura and I look at each other. Rasa reclines on her corner bed.

"Who is he that all of these beings offer him energy?" Laura wonders.

"It's like one of those fairy tales where you pick up a frog, or a dog—rescue it, take care of it, love it—and then one day you find out it's a prince, or you are granted three wishes. Whoever could know that picking up a scrawny abandoned dog and loving it all its life—that that dog is some powerful being in another realm? To me he's Kundun, but I'm beginning to see him in awe now."

Kundun continues, "Zuma has stomach problems. There is something on the base of his head or on his neck that has to do with the way she is holding him after nursing. Tell Cassidy not to lay him on his back too soon after nursing."

"Rasa, do you have any questions for me?"

"Are we getting another dog?"

"No, you get to be the only dog."

"My collar is too tight."

"Isn't her collar new?"

"Oh, I know what she means. On our last walk two little dogs that were off leash charged her growling and barking, so she thought she'd attack them. I pulled too hard and it choked her. We are going to use her harness again."

"I want you to leave earlier for the stable so I can go too."

"It's been so hot I haven't been able to leave her in the car. There isn't anywhere to park in the shade. Oh dear, our time is up already!"

Laura looks at me, "You are an extraordinary animal owner—you do know that don't you?"

"I feel so guilty for Tara being abused at her own home while in my care. I had no idea people could be so cruel and crazy. It makes me sick. It took me so long to figure out what happened and then the damage was done."

"But you don't know what Tara's karma was. Maybe you were the perfect person to have her and help her through her fear and suffering. I can't imagine anyone else loving her, caring for her and helping her so much. She could have been more abused, killed. You don't know."

"I'll try to understand that. I'm thankful she is no longer suffering. I had no idea how much time I spent taking care of her and worrying about her. I feel like I don't know what to do now I have so much time. I dedicated years to trying to keep her safe, loved and healthy. Whatever the karma was—it was my karma too."

This is the point at which I finally recognize the trajectory of Tara's health decline. It began with the rat poison. She had digestive issues continuously after that. I am convinced that the toxins in the poison caused her cancer—a hideous nerve cell destroyer causing seizures and mobility problems ultimately shutting down her ability to eat and digest food. Again she was the victim of the actions of a careless employee acting independently of any analytical thought or communication with me.

I eat lunch outside, the weather is so warm. Then I place the burgundy color paper bag decorated with cut-out hearts and miniature prints of dog paws on the willow table in front of me. I pull out the tissue paper. I unwrap the round plaster cast of Tara's foot print. It isn't a good imprint and I'm disappointed. Then I reach into the bag with both hands and place the tissue wrapped wood box on my lap. I take the paper off. It is beautiful cherry wood. When I see the black brass name plate on top, I sob, "Oh Tara!" The tears flow freely and my life feels so empty without her sweet, silly presence.

That night I lay awake on my right side facing Tara's former place on the bed. It is before dawn and my eyes are open. The moon has set and it is dark. Suddenly I see a vapor-like trail of something luminous rise from her place. It accumulates quickly into a sphere that floats a small distance above the bed. The sphere has a pattern that radiates from the center. The pattern changes like a kaleidoscope then it all vanishes.

I realize I just saw Tara!

60

I hear a loud noise at the door. It is not a dog scratching on wood or glass—it is a metal clanging racket. I wake and sit up. I look at the door and see Tara. I jump out of bed and run to the door to open it. Tara comes into the house. Her back is covered with snow. I fall onto her saying, "Oh, Tara, Tara, Tara." I hug her and kiss the top of her head. I hear her words from last autumn, "I will die in snow." I wake, "Oh, Tara, thank you for coming to visit me. I miss you so much."

Today is my appointment with Dr. Kathleen Ayl, animal grief counselor. I am going to the complimentary grief counseling included with Tara's private cremation at Guardian Animal Aftercare. I hand her a photo of Tara standing on the hill behind the house. "This is Tara."

"She is beautiful. She looks like she was painted all of those incredible colors."

"She is thirteen years old in this photo."

"Her eyes—the way she is looking at you, I can tell that you had a very deep connection."

"We had a special relationship. Right now I am struggling with so much guilt. She was abused by sadistic workmen at her own home. I didn't know they were abusing her. She wasn't safe. It was my fault—I was in charge. I didn't get it. I feel like I have soggy noodles in my head—so dense I didn't figure it out for months."

"How did you find out?"

"I had two friends visiting and one of them playfully picked up a fleece ball and threw it. Before the words, 'Stop, don't throw it,' were out of my mouth Tara dived into her crate, a look of complete terror on her face. Then five years later I hired a couple to be caretakers and they abused her. It was simply endless for this poor dog. And I didn't get it. I have so much guilt and remorse I can't sleep. I can't eat."

"Perhaps you believed that people wouldn't do things like this."

"No, I didn't. I was raised by a grandmother who was a devout Christian

Scientist. In her world everything was good. Tragic things happened in her life, but basically evil did not assault her."

"You did what you thought was the right thing to do at the time."

"I followed the advice with Tara that you gave me for Kundun to change things after he died. I washed all of the kitchen rugs and donated them to the thrift shop. I bought new rugs. I donated the blankets and towels that I used for her bedding to the shelter. Does everyone go through this guilt in the grieving process?"

"Yes. People say, 'I should've taken her to the beach.' 'I shouldn't have taken her to the beach—that's where she got sick.' 'I didn't give him all of his medications,' 'I should have changed his food,' 'I didn't take her on enough walks.'"

"I can relate to every one of those. Is it the same when a person dies?"

"Yes."

I bring Rasa with me to the stable to talk to Genji. "How are you Genji?"

"My left groin and right hip cramp all of the time—not while we are riding, but afterwards. I want to ride on a flat road. I don't mind how it is here. I'm used to the horses coming and going now. I don't pay any attention to the drama. If I move I want to be close to Mom. I want to be where people love horses. Most people here don't think of their horses as family."

"Are your feed and supplements okay?"

"I am doing okay. The nights are warmer now."

"I like coming with Mom to the stable. The fresh air makes me feel good. My house and my mom are beginning to separate. We're looking for a new home."

Laura asks, "Are you looking for a new home?"

"I think Rasa is going into my mind. I'm thinking about it, about having a place where Genji can live also."

"No one is connected to each other here," Genji states. And Genji has a good point. Each time the manager changes, people and horses leave. Other people and horses move in. In his barn in particular the overturn has been every horse twice now except Genji.

Genji touches Rasa's side with his top lip and smells her ear. Rasa growls.

"How are the little spirits?"

"I see them. They come at night and make the stars brighter. I'm afraid to move to a new stable. I may get abused. I'm not abused here. Let's get our own place. I'm upset about Mom not being happy."

"I'm still so sad about Tara. I feel so guilty about not protecting her. She wasn't safe at her own home."

"You can't keep thinking about this—it will eat you," Kundun emphatically states.

"I'm brave now. Mom healed me. You did protect me. When I died the fear all went away. I fly through the air!"

"Tara is showing me a dog-like Pegasus."

"I'm really brave. I'm in a good place. I'm not suffering now. I had to endure all of that until I learned to trust you."

"Past life," Laura intones.

"Jake and Karen were afraid of dogs."

"She is showing me Jake's leg getting mauled when he was young. He was afraid he would get mauled again."

"Zuma is eating more!" Kundun exclaims. "I am walking a lot with Tara. Keep Genji where he is. It will get better," he advises.

"I can't tell the future yet, I am still getting strong," Tara adds.

"I even worried about her in Heaven!" I look at Laura and smile.

"I worried about Maia in Heaven," Laura confesses.

"Sometimes I sleep on the bed at the end by your feet. If you stretch your feet out, you will feel me," Tara tells me. "Kundun and I see each other every day and walk together. There are waterfalls here—beautiful waterfalls."

"Do you like waterfalls?" Laura asks me.

"I love waterfalls. We had them on the land in New Mexico, and I love to hike to waterfalls and swim in the pools in Hawaii."

"You should come read me parts of a book," Genji requests. "I get lonely. I want you to come three times a week. There isn't one horse here that was here when I came."

"Yes, the dressage horses in the big barn were here."

"I want to be in a big barn with an aisle in the middle."

"Oh, Laura, a horse in one of those corrals went off its feed and had symptoms of colic. The new manager helped the owner transport it to a veterinary clinic where the horse was diagnosed with late term colic that had caused necrosis in the intestines and it had to be euthanized. Remember when

Genji said a horse died over there several months ago? Well, it just did!"

"The next time this happens remind me to ask him if it's a past event or a future event."

Rasa is panting and restless, pulling on the leash. I put her in the car. I turn Genji out in the large round turn-out pen. He rolls and rolls. Laura and I watch as he gets back on his feet and begins to gallop in half-circles along the curve of the fence closest to the barn and corrals. Laura and I walk toward her car. She begins to laugh, "He is saying, 'Are you watching me? I am running now. Do you see me?'"

"To the other horses?"

"Yes."

"That is so funny."

After I groom Genji and put him in his stall with his apples and carrots treat, I walk over to the large barn with the aisle. I wander up one side and down the other looking for empty unused stalls. There are several and there is one in particular that I think might work for Genji.

61

invite Genji, Rasa, Tara and Kundun to share wisdom they want to tell the readers of the book, things they want humans to know. We begin with Genji, "People who have horses can find pieces of themselves that are missing. But also people can take pieces of horses away—that is from abuse. When people love animals they become better people. A horse should have one person love it all its life."

"How long have you had Genji?"

"Almost fourteen years."

"How old is he?"

"He'll be seventeen in May."

"Write about rainbows. The nicer you are to animals, the more rainbows you have in your life." Genji's gaze turns toward the mountain to the east. "The little spirits are moving underground because there is something bad in the air."

I wonder if it's from the reactor in Japan, the one year anniversary of the earthquake and tsunami was a few days ago," Laura comments.

"Let's ask Bhakti what he wants to contribute for the readers," I suggest. Laura silently communicates with him for a long time.

"One incident of aggressiveness can scare you, can paralyze you. Learning to change can be difficult, but it is the best thing for you. There are stairs going up to escape the fear, but you have to trust who is helping you. It has to be someone you know. As the steps go up higher they get lighter and lighter. Kundun is helping me get there. Am I in the book?"

"Yes, Bhakti, you are!"

"It's interesting, isn't it, how each animal has such a different experience after death," I state, as I reflect on the beautiful image Bhakti has given us.

"They always show us themselves in their animal form, I wonder if they have other forms in Heaven?" Laura asks curiously.

Rasa speaks next, "It is important to pay attention and watch animals.

Inside us is a deep knowing. Our lives become deeper and richer when our person becomes deeper and richer. Some of our sadness and illnesses come so our person will learn to love more deeply and go the extra distance to make us well, to heal us."

Laura asks, "Is there more that you want to say?"

"Dogs have a life with each other. We communicate with each other. Our relationship with each other reflects our person's relationship with us. Be more present in life rather than confused in the head. Animals miss their friends when they die. Animals cry inside. Animals have feelings. Some animals fight out of fear, not anger."

Laura asks, "What do you mean?"

"Tara smelled bad. It scared me."

"After her seizure?"

"She always smelled bad."

"Rasa attacked Tara all of her life. It's a relief to not have to deal with it anymore."

"Maybe she smelled from fear," Laura offers.

Tara joins us, "Love is expansive and when you die it continues to fill you and take care of you. People need to know that they can't tell how grateful an animal is, but every step you take with them, the animal recognizes that and is grateful. When people cry over their pets, the animals don't want them to cry. Sometimes wild and scared animals need nature to feel free but need to be contained to feel safe."

Kundun expresses, "Sorrow with animals can be so deep, but if you open yourself up and learn from it—it's worth it. Do it again. Have another animal. It is like playing chess. You need a lot of focused attention having a pet. Life is like that. There is fate, but there are also moves that you choose. When you feel like you've lost, just play another game and get better."

"What is chess?" Rasa asks.

Laura explains it to her silently.

"Does it make you angry?"

"Only some people if they lose," I answer.

"Is there anything you'd like them to comment on that's in the book?"

"Yes, that horrendous treatment by Dr. Monroe, what happened?"

Kundun responds, "He crushed my spine, which set off antibodies fighting each other. He has the ability to be thorough, but was distracted. It's okay, I'm happy. That man learned a deep lesson. He was afraid to work and cancelled many days."

Because I became fascinated by my higher self after Tara went to me/her after she died, I ask Tara, "Do you continue to see my higher self?"

"Yes, by the waterfall at the Sacred Pool. I also see sparks of you connecting to your higher self when you write."

"Is it possible to connect more with my higher self and integrate my higher self with myself in this realm?"

"Of course it is. You do every day—every time you write, meditate, walk. The more aware you are of your thoughts, the more your higher self can guide you."

"Picture yourself walking with me and I'll take you on a journey. Drink less wine. Alcohol closes out the angels. Take Tai Chi," Kundun adds.

"The best way to connect with your higher self is to go on a walk with me!" Rasa exclaims. I've learned a lot from Mom and a lot from the book."

"What have you learned?" Laura asks.

"Life is not what you think."

62

Laura and I arrive at the same time to visit Genji. He sees us get out of our cars. We walk to his corral which faces the parking area. After saying hello we walk around to the end of the barn and walk along the aisle which has stalls facing it on each side. Genji's is the third stall on the right. He meets us at his stall door. I slide it open and put on his halter. Outside he grabs mouth after mouthful of grass that hasn't been mowed yet between the two barns.

"What do you want to talk about today?"

"Genji, how do you like being in the big barn in your new stall?"

"The other horses in this barn have good moms and they have happy lives. It isn't noisy—I sleep better."

"Remember how he didn't like the wind blowing through the other barn? This stall has a solid door and the shed-row barn has wire gates. He also likes the cross-ties while I groom and saddle him. The hitching rail always seemed to bother him, or the activity around it did.

"When we were riding a week ago we saw a mountain lion. It wasn't a big one and it kept trotting on the trail in front of us. It wasn't that far away, maybe one hundred feet. There was a slight hill with a curve and it vanished. I looked but I couldn't see it on either side."

"Oh Genji, what did you think when you saw the mountain lion?"

"The lion said, 'You aren't supposed to see me.' I told the lion, it's okay, my mom loves animals."

Laura and I laugh at this unexpected interchange between predator and prey. Genji is full of energy as Ernesto fires up the weed-trimmer to cut the grass. He prances and pulls as we walk toward the large round turn-out pen. I decide that he needs a turn-out right now. Laura and I watch Genji roll and roll in the soft sand. He gets back up on his feet, shakes from head to tail and begins to gallop in huge circles around the perimeter. His long mane and tail fly in the wind he creates. He bucks and when he stops he does a kung fu kick backwards with each hind leg.

"This is the most energetic turn-out he has had for ages!"

"Do you want to talk to Kundun?"

"Yes! What are you doing Kundun?"

"I take Tara for a walk every day. Sometimes we lay in the sun, or on your bed!"

"Tara is here."

"I miss you Tara."

"I miss you too."

"Tara is getting used to being petted by women, men and children," Kundun tells us.

"Every day I sit with you at the waterfall and we work to get rid of the fears imprinted on me."

I visualize my higher self with her as we heal the fears that my mortal self could not assuage while she was with me in this realm. The mystical nature of this is elusive, but it is very healing to me to perceive the continuation between realms. When I talk to Tara and tell her goodnight before I sleep, I always say, "See you at the waterfall." And now I discover that is where we are.

"I take Tara to the clouds and we practice being foggy, being clear, being foggy, being clear. Whenever I see Ganesha I ask him to smooth out Tara's obstacles."

"Genji, did the little spirits come back up out of the earth?"

"Yes, and they brought many, many crystals with them. They are putting crystals in our hooves. But you have to be here to get the crystals." Genji's hooves have never looked as healthy as they do now, which makes me wonder about the little spirits and their healing crystals. "The little spirits have a crystal they want to give you, but they don't know how to get it to you."

Laura leaves. I put Genji's halter back on and we walk to the barn. I groom him, saddle him and we take a trail ride. The sky is intermittent fog and sun. A breeze blows in from the ocean. The air smells clean and feels cool. Hills are verdant from the April rains. On the flattest stretch of dirt road Genji gaits the smoothest, fastest largo he's done for a long time. I think I finally have my horse back.

aura arrives at the house. Rasa enthusiastically barks a greeting from the porch as she drives in then she runs around to the kitchen door.

"Rasa, how are you?" I ask.

"I am feeling really good in my body. I want long walks so I get tired. I saw Kundun ahead of us at the beach, but when we got there he was gone."

I describe what happened while I was in bed a few nights ago, "I was lying on my back looking at the window which is beyond the foot of the bed. I sleep on three pillows so my head was elevated. The lights were off and the room was dark. Suddenly an explosive brilliant white light filled the window. At first I thought it was a firework then realized that with a large California pepper tree outside the window it wouldn't look like it was so close plus there was no sound. The screen rattled just a little and the light began to coruscate with geometric rays coming from the center. It vanished as I sat up and reached for Rasa. Was that Kundun?"

"That is the Crystal Angel Goddess that you used to know in the cave."

I look at Laura and shake my head no, "Maybe Rasa knew her there, but I didn't."

"Does Tara know the Crystal Angel Goddess?" Laura asks.

"The Crystal Angel Goddess is who fixed her brain."

"Wow, and I got to see her! Rasa, I'm leaving for a week. I'm going to Santa Fe to Alan's eighth grade graduation. You are going to Kelly's while I'm gone."

"I want to stay at home."

"Brandy can't come this week, but she will stay with you in June. Tara, how are you doing?"

"There are windows where I am. I traveled to the center of the earth where it's hot. There is a whole other world there. The Crystal Angel Goddess lives between there and here. Don't worry about the animals and leaving, right now they are okay. I am playing a lot here. I let things go over my head and have to trust my intuition about when to duck. I am so proud of how the book is coming now. Your posture and the way you are carrying yourself is much better. I enjoy talking together every day."

"Kundun, what are you doing?"

"I'm riding the waves—not waves of water. They are waves of air. They are waves of creation and magnetism—waves into your soul. I am living as if I am a fast moving particle. I'm in between visualization and actualization. Whatever you want, I can help you with attaining it.

"The magic of Kundun in body may come back some day. I'm still figuring out how I want to look. I want to be unique."

"How will I know?"

"You will see a dog and think—I have to have that dog!"

BIBLIOGRAPHY

Abney, Don. Catahoula History. http://www.abneycatahoulas.com/history. php. (accessed September 2012).

"Bear Dance comes to Ojai." *Ojai Valley News*, November 6, 2009.

De la Guerra y Pacheco, Chapter 1.5, E Clampus Vitus. Historic Plaque. October 2009.

"DFG issues report on bear killing," *Ojai Valley News*, October 23, 2009.

Dog Fancy. Breed Bites. July 2010.

Halsey, Richard. Director, California Chaparral Institute. Lecture. October 6, 2012.

Keller, Ed. Professor, Earth Science. UCSB. Lecture. November 5, 2011.

McCall, Lynne, and Rosalind Perry, comp. California's Chumash Indians. EZ Nature Books. 1996.

Rubens, Connie. The Barb Horse. *Paso Fino Horse World*, May 1999.

Schuhmacher, Stephen, and Gert Woerner, ed. The Encyclopedia of Eastern Philosophy and Religion. Shambala. 1994.

Shikibu, Murasaki. The Tale of Genji. Edward G. Seidensticker, trans. Alfred A. Knopf. 1992.

Stinchfield, Laura. "Pet Psychic." *Ojai Valley News*, March 18, 2011.

"Warden and the bear," *Ojai Valley News*, October 30, 2009.

Villalobos, Dr. Alice. "Soft Tissue Sarcomas." Pawspice & Animal Oncology Consultation Service. October 2, 2010.

———. Oncology Outlook. *Veterinary Product News*, November 1999.

CPSIA information can be obtained
at www.ICGtesting.com
Printed in the USA
FSOW01n2039250817
38022FS